AIDS
AND BIOLOGICAL WARFARE

WILLIAM CAMPBELL DOUGLASS, MD

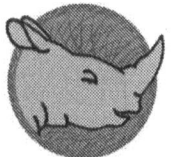

Rhino Publishing, S.A.
Panama City
Republic of Panama

AIDS
AND BIOLOGICAL WARFARE

ISBN 9962-636-07-8

Cover illustration by
Ron Lindahn
and
Alex Manyoma (alex@3dcity.com).

Please, visit Rhino's website for other publications from
Dr. William Campbell Douglass
www.rhinopublish.com

Dr. Douglass' "Real Health" alternative medical newsletter
is available at www.realhealthnews.com

RHINO PUBLISHING, S.A.
World Trade Center
Panama, Republic of Panama

Voicemail/Fax
International: + 416-352-5126
North America: 888-317-6767

Dedication

This book is dedicated to Robert Strecker, M.D. without whose brilliance and courage none of us today would have the slightest idea what really happened to cause the current AIDS epidemic.

And to the memory of Theodore A. Strecker, L.L.B., who was one of the first political casualties in this war against the dark forces that would destroy western civilization.

Acknowledgements

My debt to Patricia Vanderslice, Doyle Payne and the world's best newscaster, Robert, is beyond future payment. To these "favorite moles" I would like to add my thanks to **all subscribers to *my* Newsletter** who have sent me "hot" material from all over the United States and all corners of the world.

Howard Pearson saved us from grammatical, syntactical and tautological disaster.

We are grateful to Nick Lester for helping us "bring it together" and insisting that we "give 'em a little hope" at the end.

One shy person without whose expertise and energy and intelligence the book could not have been written does not want her name mentioned, so I will simply say thanks to BC's good friend, BON.

My thanks to Ed O'Neal for his editing and expertise in the publishing field which got the project off the ground and into book form.

Dr. John Seale has generously shared his extensive knowledge and ideas, and Vivian Bird has helped enormously with his "cuttings," as the English call them, from the British press.

Thanks also to Lib, Leah and Lee for doing so much of the basic "scut work" without which a book could not be published.

Contents

Foreword

Still thou art blest, compared wi' me!
The present only toucheth thee:
But Och! I backwards cast my e'e,
On prospects dear! An'forward, though I canna see,
I guess an'fear!

                   - Robert Burns, "To a Mouse," 1785

We have been robbed of our defenses like a crusading knight without his armor. But even worse, like a disarmed knight, we have no javelin, bow or mace to confront the enemy hordes.

We are a naked species.

Our most vigorous and productive age group, from 20 to 40 years old, is widely infected with an incurable disease. If you haven't begun to panic then you simply don't understand the magnitude of the problem. Maynard Jackson, former mayor of Atlanta, Georgia, said[1] that he believes the epidemic is "almost a biblical pestilence." Recent reports from Georgia, only tenth in this national AIDS die-off, are revealing and terrifying.

Dr. Brian Williams of the Public Health Department reported that "in the first half of 1988 there was *one reported death per day* from AIDS. By the end of the year the rate had gone to *one and a half deaths per day.*" Williams noted that there were twice as many cases in 1986 as there had been in the previous five years.

"It's out of control," said James Alley, also from the Georgia Department of Health. *Five of every 1,000 Georgians have been infected,* based on information gathered at blood banks, from pre-marital testing and from the military.

---

1 *Atlanta Journal*, 1212/88.

"The members of the fastest-growing group are not adults," said Dr. Andre Nahmias,[2] professor of pediatrics at Emory University. "They are children."

"At this point," Dr. Alley said, "what we are trying to avoid is mass hysteria." You can forget about the population implosion. We are facing a population implosion of unprecedented dimensions. The next 10 years may reveal the most incredible "massacre by nature" in the history of the world. There will be a true generation gap: the old at one end of the age spectrum; and the very young at the other; and no one in between.

Children are amazing. They can make a game or joke out of the most horrible and grotesque of situations.

"Ring around the rosey, a pocket full of posies, ashes, ashes, we all fall down," was a children's verse describing the worst plague in recorded history, the Black Death of the middle ages. The typical little red boils of the plague were surrounded by a red ring ("ring around the rosey"). Infected people smelled terrible so the victims carried flowers in their pockets to disguise the odor ("a pocket full of posies"). Ashes were mixed with water to serve as an ointment ("ashes, ashes"). The dying would, as humans are prone to do, just keep going until the end, and then drop dead on the street ("we all fall down").

By the end of 1962 the government had its 4-H club to blame for the AIDS epidemic: one had to be a homosexual, a Haitian, a heroin addict or a hemophiliac who got AIDS from a blood transfusion, to be in the "risk groups."

The government embarked on a tragic course of disinformation and outright lies to the American people that have now put us in a position where the AIDS epidemic may be unstoppable.

---

2 *Gwinnett Daily News*, 12/1/88

Ward Cates of the U.S. Centers for Disease Control said: "Anyone who has the least ability to look into the future can already see the potential for this disease being much worse than anything mankind has seen before."

The World Future Society predicts that 50 million lives will be lost throughout the world in the 1990s from the AIDS epidemic. This will exceed the toll of the Black Plague of the Middle Ages, according to the World Future Society report.

The report is the grimmest of many forecasts by the Society, which appeared in the November-December edition of its magazine, *The Futurist*. It said millions of Americans may become ill with AIDS and the economic cost to the nation will be $66 billion.[3]

The World Future Society estimate of 50 million lives lost by 1990 is probably very, very low. The World Health Organization has predicted at least that many cases of AIDS in Africa alone.

The medical establishment told us that the AIDS virus was "fragile." The virus is in fact one of the hardiest viruses known to man and will live on a dry petri dish in the open air for 10 days. The AIDS virus can withstand a concentration of chlorine ten times what it takes to kill bacteria.

The government assured us that AIDS is not insect-borne. As you will see, insect transmission of the disease through mosquitoes, ticks, biting flies, bed bugs, etc., is almost certain.

Perhaps the most startling and disturbing attempt at disinformation by government spokesmen was the monkey bite theory of transmission of AIDS. This is not only false, but doctors such as Robert Gallo and Myron Essex, who are perpetrating this story, are fully aware that it is genetically impossible for the African

---

3   *AP,* 10/19188.

9

monkey to have started the AIDS epidemic. We will go into more detail in Chapter 4.

They told us back in 1981 that only a small percentage of people infected with the AIDS virus would actually come down with the AIDS disease. It is now admitted that probably *everyone* who contracts the AIDS virus will eventually die of the disease.

There has been a constant mantra that "You can't catch AIDS from casual contact." The evidence is clear, however, that AIDS is not a typical sexually transmitted disease; it can be contracted through abrasions of the skin and may very well be contracted through saliva. The term "casual contact" does not appear in any medical dictionary and is being used as a smoke screen to allay the fears of the American people. Because of the hardiness of the AIDS virus, it is certainly possible, if not certain, that AIDS can be transmitted through fomites. Fomites are inanimate objects such as towels, handkerchiefs, dishes, bedding, etc. It is interesting to note that the Pasteur Institute, which treated the movie star, Rock Hudson, thoroughly fumigated the room and burned all the bedding and bed clothes of Hudson when he left. The Pasteur Institute is where the AIDS virus was discovered, and they apparently have some question about fomite transfer of AIDS. Our government ridicules anyone who makes such a suggestion.

A government spokesman told us early in the epidemic that it was difficult for females to catch the virus. They had absolutely no scientific studies to back up such a statement, and we now know that females catch the virus just as easily as males.

It is truly astounding that in the face of this rapidly spreading plague, officials remain adamant against routine testing for AIDS. The government also holds steadfast on the subject of quarantine, although quarantine is the only technology we have at this point to protect the American public from the AIDS epidemic.

Casting a Bewildering Shadow

New research reveals that the AIDS virus, which once appeared to be a manageable single entity, is a complex family of rapidly mutating viruses that, like a clever enemy, can constantly change its weaponry, its camouflage, its defenses, and even its targets in the body.

As a result of mutations in the AIDS virus there are thousands of slightly different forms, including many that have acquired new specialized abilities to be transmitted, to infect different tissues, to invade the immune system and to resist drug treatments—a biological weapon system of unparalleled capability.

The Los Alamos National Laboratory report reveals that the AIDS virus mutates at least five times faster than the influenza virus which has always been considered the fastest mutating virus.

The flu virus has taken 50 years to evolve as much as the AIDS virus has evolved in the last 10 years, the Los Alamos study revealed. The Los Alamos finding "casts a bewildering shadow" over the prospects of a reliable diagnosis, an effective treatment or a preventive vaccine.[4]

Dr. Gerald Myers of the Los Alamos laboratory said that his evidence supports the view that the AIDS virus has only recently come into existence, "having arisen from some *unknown ancestor.*" (As you will see from this book, the ancestors are *clearly* known.)

Dr. Myers points out the futility of trying to develop an AIDS vaccine. Also the variations make it probable that in the future the AIDS tests will not work. They will not detect the variations of the virus.[5]

Dr. Jonathan Mann, testifying before the Presidential AIDS Commission on April 19th, 1988, said that "hundreds of millions" of people worldwide may contract

---

4 *Washington Post,* 9/7/87
5 Ibid.

11

AIDS in the near future. "Unless a curative treatment or a preventive vaccine is developed," he said, *"the AIDS virus will perpetuate itself."* Mann said that he has a "somber view" of the future because a treatment or preventive is "unlikely' in the near future. This grim announcement was found at the bottom of page six of the *Atlanta Journal*.[6]

To understand AIDS one must understand the entire mosaic of the current attack against western civilization. We will cover the bio-chemical aspect of this continuing war with emphasis on the biological. We will discuss the psycho-political threat to show that the attack against us is indeed *integrated, organized and carefully planned.*

We have been criticized, even by fellow conservatives, for stating that the AIDS virus is man-made in a laboratory and probably done for subversive reasons. The critics say, "There's an old African saying that you don't worry how the lion got in your house, you worry about how you're going to get him out." To which we replied, "You'd better learn how the lion got in the house, or you're going to end up with more lions in the house—and some tigers too."

To understand AIDS you must understand virology and genetics. So there will be a chapter explaining, in laymen's terms, how these things work. The reason that scientists such as Robert Gallo of the National Cancer Institute and Myron Essex of Harvard Medical School can distort and actually lie to the American people is because they know that the average man on the street has no idea what virology and genetics are all about. Clear understanding of the basics of these sciences will enable you to see that the American people have been deliberately lied to by the very people who are supposed to lead us out of this AIDS wilderness.

---

6 *Atlanta Journal*, 4/19/88, p. 6.

We will discuss vaccinations because the government is going to waste tens of millions of dollars pursuing a type of preventive medicine which has never worked, does not work now, and never will work for AIDS or any other disease.

There will be a chapter on heterosexuals and how they interrelate in the spread of AIDS.

To give the reader some historical perspective, there is a chapter on the history of plagues and how, in spite of modern medicine, those plagues continue to this very day. The AIDS plague is different in that there is no known cure, the mode of transmission is still open to question and no treatment is in sight. In the plagues of old at least 10 percent of the population would survive and continue to propagate the human race. The AIDS pandemic is far more serious than any plague in history because, as far as we know, no one survives.

During the TB epidemic of the 19th and early 20th centuries, the optimistic pronouncements sounded eerily like the present ones from government and scientific authorities concerning advances in the treatment of AIDS. Authors in 1910 said ". . . the medical profession has acquired such a grasp of thc essential facts connected with the disease that the bulk of the scientific work which was necessary to make the eradication of tuberculosis possible, within no distant date, has been accomplished. We know how to prevent and how to cure tuberculosis, and the statesmen must be made to realize that the eradication of the disease lies in their hands."[7]

Lloyd George in 1911 said: "Men who have devoted a great deal of attention to the subject . . . are full of bright hopes that they can stamp it out."[8]

---

7 Latham & Garland, **The Conquest of Consumption,** 1910.

8 Hansard, **Fifth Series,** 1911.

Having the advantage of hindsight we can see that this was way off the mark. A true cure of tuberculosis with chemotherapeutic agents, INH and streptomycin, did not come along until 30 years later. It is not unreasonable to expect that it will take 30 years or longer to find a cure or preventive for AIDS and, by that time, the human race may be extinct.

Because of the horror of AIDS in children and the alarmingly rapid increase in this disease among our young people, there is a chapter on AIDS and children.

The World Health Organization has played a central role in this disease. The exact way in which the World Health Organization interfaces with the National Cancer Institute and the National Institute of Health is not clear. But what is clear is that the relationship somehow led to the AIDS epidemic in Africa. It is no secret that agents of the Soviet government have been working in our "top secret" biological warfare laboratories for many years, thanks to the "glasnost" of Richard Nixon during his presidency. We will probably never know how these agents engineered this attack on the free world beyond the fact that the situation in Africa, Brazil and Haiti where the World Health Organization introduced AIDS, speaks for itself.

As AIDS is only one of many, many forms of possible biological attack, we devote a chapter to biological weapons in general. We will quote Soviet generals who have openly admitted that the war against the free world will be fought with biological weapons. The Soviets have never failed to tell us exactly what they are going to do. The problem has been to get our leaders and the American people to believe that they are going to do what they say they are going to do.

The American military is finally awakening to this devastating and shocking threat of biological warfare.

14

Plans are now afoot to protect the American military, but *there are no plans to do anything to protect the civilian population of the United States. In other words, you are on your own.*

Prevention of AIDS, i.e., condoms, education and changing human behavior, the holy trinity of AIDS prevention at the present time, will be discussed in detail. None of these approaches have been or will be successful, and a continuation of this misguided approach will lead to the death of our great nation.

Because of the importance of identification and quarantine of the AIDS-infected, we will devote a chapter to explain the history of quarantine and why it is absolutely essential to isolate any AIDS patient who shows any mental or physical signs of the disease. It would in fact be better to isolate, i.e. quarantine, all AIDS-infected people but, as the government has dragged its feet for so long, that would probably be politically impossible.

The message is clear: *We are in World War III.* If we do not treat it as an all-out war, we will lose not only our freedoms but our lives.

* * *

"Grandpa, what was a Singles Bar?"

"A Singles Bar was a place where young men and women met in the evening after work."

"Why?"

"Well, they were looking for a little action."

"What's 'action', Grandpa?" The little girl licked her frozen broccoli stick.

Grandpa was one of the last of the great smokers. He tapped out the burned ashes from his pipe. Have to give it up soon, he mused. He loved his pipe but it wasn't worth a jail sentence. The new "smoke-out" law provided harsh penalties for offenders. How ridiculous, he thought, after 98 percent of the population had died of The virus the bureaucrats run around looking for smokers.

15

"Action means they would have a few drinks and then get together at his or her house." Or sometimes *his* house or *his* house, he thought gloomily.

Grandpa attempted to divert the conversation. You can't explain sex to a seven-year-old. "Would you like another frozen broccoli stick?" How does she eat that stuff? What ever happened to popsicles? He jammed his pipe into his shirt pocket.

"Why did the Singles Bar go away, Grandpa?"

How did she know about singles bars? he mused. The last one closed before she was born. What a question.

Grandpa scowled down at her round face with broccoli juice, like moss, encircling her mouth. "How did you know about singles bars? That was before you were born—what do you care anyway?"

She flushed and stared at the ground. He cursed himself for losing his temper. "I'm sorry, honey. But why are you asking me about such things?" He stroked her blond hair.

"Well, Daddy says that's what killed everybody."

"No, honey, the bars didn't kill anybody. It was a virus. Some people got it from doing some things they shouldn't have done. It took a long time to get sick. Before they got sick they infected dozens of others and those people, not knowing they were sick, infected still more people.

"By the time the first ones died, millions of our young people were infected. And then they started dying by the thousands." His face was damp with sweat. The little girl was transfuxed.

"Your Uncle Bob and Aunt Ethel died of The virus and then your big brother, Tom. Thousands, tens of thousands, and then millions died–a whole generation, gone."

He looked down the long empty main street. His house, a mansion now decayed into a ramshackle shell of

16

peeling paint and windows without glass, like the eye sockets of a human skull, was at the end of Main Street adjoining what used to be the small city college.

The night's bodies had been picked up from the street earlier but the stench of diseased flesh lingered. The smoke from the crematory across town spiraled lazily upward. He had told his granddaughter they were burning trash.

"Am I going to die, Grandpa?" Her eyes were wide and searching.

"No, darling, you're not. You and your generation are going to have to rebuild this country."

"I don't understand."

"No, sweetheart, I know you don't."

He could see the smoke police in their black car driving slowly toward them. He took her by the hand and turned toward the decaying house. Pipe tobacco aroma carries a long way. You can't be too careful.

* * * * * *

Is this little story improbable fiction? The frozen broccoli sticks are, hopefully. The Smoke Police, maybe. But the AIDS epidemic promises to become the greatest natural disaster since the Great Flood.

Some of the chapters at first appear unconnected to the subject of AIDS. But you will see as you progress through the book that the story of the ancient plagues has startling and very disturbing parallels with today's epidemic. The biological warfare chapter is apropos because AIDS ~s biological warfare. The question of quarantine is of the utmost importance, and we have devoted a chapter to it because historically quarantine has been the only way to prevent the rapid spread of an infection when there is no known cure and the mode of transmission is not entirely understood.

One must see the AIDS plague in the entire context of the attack against western civilization which includes not only AIDS, but drugs, pornography through such devices as "sex education," and the incredible peace offensive which has convinced most Americans that the Russian leaders are more trustworthy than ours!

Not all of these subjects will be covered in this book (they will be in a subsequent book), but we have covered enough of the overall mosaic of psychological and biological war to put the AIDS epidemic in proper perspective.

We have presented a very bleak and discouraging picture which may tempt you to believe that things are hopeless. Although the situation is serious, it is not hopeless; but the American people need to be shocked into a sense of reality concerning this epidemic. A nation and its people cannot take intelligent action against a threat until they clearly understand the magnitude of the threat.

We suggest that you "grit your teeth" and read the terrible truth. In the last chapter we will outline what can and must be done to reverse this rapidly-advancing viral plague.

Chapter 1
The AIDS Pandemic—History Repeats

If Stone Age man had left behind a written history of the Mesolithic period, we would surely know that plagues have been part and parcel of the human condition since 10,000 B.C. At that time man began domesticating plants and animals. Communities developed and with them the crowded living conditions that are fertile ground for disease and plague.

We do have clear evidence of bubonic plague as long ago as 1100 B.C. The Philistines defeated an army of Hebrews at Eben-ezer and captured the sacred ark of the Covenant. The ark was carried triumphantly to Ashdod near the Mediterranean and then the trouble began: "The hand of the Lord was against the city with a very great destruct80n: and He smote them into the city, both small and great, and they had emerods[1] in their secret parts" (*I Samuel*, 5:9).

The definition of "emerods" is not at all clear. Literally translated it means "hemorrhoids." As the Philistines were attacked with a devastating visitation of these emerods it seems hardly likely that this was a plague of hemorrhoids. Taking another meaning of the word, which was "mound," would indicate that they were indeed suffering the bubonic plague. In the Bible God is said to have smitten his enemies "in the hinder parts."[2] The emerods or buboes of plague appear in the armpits, under the jaw and "at the secret parts," meaning the groin

---

1 Hastings, **Dictionary of the Bible.**; and Preuss, Medizin in Talmud.
2 **Psalms** LXXVIII (66).

area. Granting that we are indeed referring to swellings in the private parts with the word emerods, the only disagreement is whether these swellings were in the "hinder" or the "front end" of the body. History will always be imprecise.

The Philistines hastily took the ark to Ashdod, and with them they also carried the plague. They then took it to Ekron and the plague followed. The Philistines could only conclude that the Hebrew God was taking vengeance upon them. Terrified, they appealed to their priests for instruction.

The priests advised them to place the ark on a newly-made cart to be drawn by two milk cows. They would be set loose, and the cattle, unguided, would reveal to them the truth by the direction in which the cart was taken. If the cattle drew the cart toward the enemy Hebrew town of Beth-shemesh then this would signify that the Lord of Israel was on the side of the Hebrews and all was lost. If the cattle went the other way it would signify that all the suffering had simply been a coincidence and was not related to their defeating the Hebrews. On the cart was a great gold offering to the gods.

One day the farmers of Beth-shemesh looked up from their task of harvesting their wheat and, not believing their eyes, wiped away the sweat to see a most remarkable sight. A newly-made cart creaked into the field carrying the ark of the Covenant and a great amount of gold. The cart stopped by a great stone and the exultant farmers quickly unloaded the precious ark and gold onto the stone, and then burned the cart and cattle as an offering to the Lord. The ark had returned!

But the celebrations and offerings to God quickly stopped, because the magnificent ark also brought the bubonic plague: "And he smote the men of Beth-shemesh, because they had looked into the ark of the Lord, even He smote of the people *fifty thousand and three score and ten*

20

men: and the people lamented, because the Lord had smitten many of the people with a great slaughter" (*I Samuel* 6:19). (It must be understood that 50,070 victims of a plague in the sparsely populated world at that time was an incredible devastation.)

Historians have not appreciated the importance of epidemics in the history of various military conquests. Many historic military victories for which generals have gotten credit really should be credited to much smaller living entities such as Yersenia pestis, Cholera vibrio, measles and typhus. This neglect of the importance of infectious diseases in conquests is partially due to historians being governed by their own experience with infections. They live among populations where relatively high levels of immunity to familiar infections have tended to dampen epidemic outbreaks and cause them to be self-limiting. So historians are prone to discount as exaggeration any reports of massive die-offs from infectious disease during various military battles. They fail to understand the profound difference between a disease breaking out among experienced populations with immunity and the utter devastation that the same infection would cause on a community which had had no acquired immunity to that particular disease. Because of a lack of interest and understanding of the pivotal importance of epidemics during conquest, historians have all but ignored the military significance of plagues.

We must understand the past if we are to understand the present. Without some understanding of the cataclysmic effects that infectious diseases have had we are not able to get an overall picture of where we are today on this disastrous continuum of man's constant battle with disease and its intermingling with man's battle against himself. It would have been utterly impossible, for instance, for Cortez and his band of marauders to have conquered the highly religious and fanatically dedicated

21

Aztecs of Mexico without his great secret weapon—smallpox. In Peru, history was repeated when Pizarro's little band of roughnecks conquered the Incas with crude weapons and a numerically inferior force, but with a secret weapon: smallpox. In fact, the reigning emperor himself died of smallpox while on campaign. His designated heir also died, leaving no legitimate successor. Because of the breakdown in leadership due to the disease, civil war ensued and Pizarro with his brigands was able to enter Cuzco, the capital, plunder its treasure and take over the nation with practically no military resistance.

Even more devastating than the epidemic's effect on the bodies of the Incas and the Aztecs was the effect that it had on their minds and morality. It seemed perfectly obvious that these men who did not contract the disease were being favored by the gods, and therefore resistance was useless. It also became evident that their religion was superior to the native religion. This new God was far superior in that the disease only affected the natives and not the conquerors. This belief was, of course, reinforced by the priests who also sincerely felt that God was on their side. Consequently the Inca and Aztec religions quickly disappeared.

As Professor William H. McNeill has stated concerning the impact of disease on the invasion: "The extraordinary ease of Spanish conquest and the success a few hundred men had in securing control of vast areas and millions of persons is unintelligible on any other basis."

It is extremely important that this disease continuum and its remarkable effect on human history be understood by modern man because now, *for the first time in history, man is technological) equipped to use this awesome biological force for conquest.* It would have been impossible, as we have stated, for Pizarro and Cortez to have made their remarkable conquests without the help of "natural biological war." It is likewise highly unlikely that the disorganized, highly inefficient communist

22

endeavor to take over the world could succeed today without first demoralizing the American people morally and through disease.

The course of Chinese history and its battles was undoubtedly influenced because we know that smallpox was prevalent as early as 1000 B.C. In 1700 B.C., the Egyptians were plagued with various infections which greatly affected their civilization. Most of these infections were treated by the Egyptian doctors with the feces of donkeys. Ramses V was found to have an eruption at the groin area which would indicate that he had plague.

In the time of David it was said that 70,000 perished *in one day*. It is hard to imagine, even with our understanding of microbiology, what pestilence could have caused such a devastation. However, with modern technology, it would certainly be possible to kill 10 times 70,000 in one day with an attack of botulism toxin or a genetically altered, antibiotic-resistant pneumonic plague organism.

In the age of Hippocrates the record clearly reveals many epidemics similar to those of the present day including malaria, typhoid fever, malta fever, mumps, scarlet fever, diphtheria, typhoid, cholera and, of course, plague.

One of the first recorded epidemics which affected the outcome of war was the Athenian epidemic during the Peloponesian wars which was described in the second book of the history of Thucydides, 50Q B.C. In the summer of 430 B.C. large armies were camped in Attica, the hinterland around Athens. Consequently the people of the countryside swarmed into Athens, creating very crowded conditions. The Plague of Athens, probably typhus, had a profound effect on history. The citizens were seized rapidly with headache, red eyes, inflammation of the tongue, sneezing and cough; then came acute intestinal symptoms with vomiting, diarrhea and excessive thirst. This was usually followed by delirium with the patient usually dying in about nine days.

Because of this pestilence, Pericles did not attempt to expel the enemy who was ravaging Attica. Athenian life was completely demoralized with anarchy and extreme lawlessness. As Thucydides said, "They saw HOW sudden was the change of fortune in the case both of those who were prosperous and suddenly died, and of those who before had nothing but, any moment, were in possession of the property of others."

Although Athens was totally devastated and helpless, the Peloponesians left Attica quickly, not out of fear of the Athenians, who were locked up in their cities, but because they feared death from whatever disease God had wrought upon the Athenians. The Greeks in turn lost their battle with the Peloponesian fleet along the Peloponesian coast because they were simply too sick to carry out their objectives. It is believed that this epidemic, also called the "Plague of Thucydides," was typhus fever. But it may have been smallpox.

In 396 B.C., less than 40 years after the epidemics at Attica, the Carthagenians were devastated by an epidemic of smallpox. The importance of this epidemic and its effect on the consequent history of the world cannot be over-emphasized. Because of the plague, Carthage was prevented from controlling Sicily and from conquering Rome. Without the pox, superiority in the earlier campaigns might well have resulted in the civilization of Rome being supplanted by the superior civilization of Carthage—an event that would have profoundly affected all history, including ours. It might, in fact, have resulted in a commercial civilization being developed thousands of years before ours. Such is the power of biological warfare, whether intentional or unintentional.

The crusaders brought many of these devastating diseases from the Middle East back to Europe. It is likely that the sad fate of the army of Frederick Barbarosa was caused, not by his enemies, but by smallpox.

The conquest of Mexico was probably as much influenced by one shipload of Negroes from Narvaez than all of Cortez' troops. The ship landed and the crew infected the populace with smallpox, thus causing the death of three million Indians. So Negro slaves played a very important part in the conquest of Mexico for which due notice has not been given by historians.[3]

The bacterium called anthrax (which is a darling of the current sorcerers in the biological warfare laboratories) has a reputation for changing human history. At the time of the reign of Nero (about 50 B.C.) a plague occurred which, according to Tacitus, was "extraordinarily destructive." "Slaves as well as citizens died," according to Schnurrer, "and many who had mourned a beloved victim died themselves with such rapidity that they were carried to the same pyre as those they had mourned."

A little over a hundred years later anthrax was influential in the Hun invasion of the west. The Huns were attempting to escape anthrax and thus proceeded to Europe with 40,000 horses, 30,000 men and 100,000 cattle.

Only 85 years later in 165 A.D. the "Plague of Antonius" struck Europe. This particular plague of smallpox caused a complete abandonment of many Italian villages which then fell into ruin. The disease was so devastating that the war against Marcomanni had to be postponed. Four years later in 169 A.D., when it was felt that the pestilence had receded, the war was resumed. Many of the warriors were found dead on the field without wounds, having died from the epidemic that had indeed not left. The emperor Marcus Aurelius had contracted the disease and died in seven days. The mortality and social disruption was so great that it completely de-

---

3   Zinsser, **Rats, Lice and History,** Little, Brown & Co., Boston, 1934.

moralized Rome politically, socially and militarily. The disease again broke out in 189 A.D. and "there arose the greatest plague of any I know of. Often there were two thousand deaths a day in Rome" (Ammianus Marcellinus).

The Roman Empire breathed a sigh of relief as this pestilence passed, but their relief was short. Fifty years later the Plague of St. Cyprian hit. It swept over the entire known world from Egypt to Scotland. This additional plague left the Roman Empire almost at the mercy of its enemies. The Germanic tribes were invading Gaul and the near East. The far eastern provinces were being attacked by the Goths, and the Parthians were conquering Mesopotamia. The terror was palpable, and people were seeing phantoms hovering over the houses of those about to fall sick. St. Cyprian made many conversions to Christianity by exorcising these evil spirits. This "plague of Cyprian," as it was called, was apparently bubonic plague. Haesser said: "Men crowded into the large cities; only the nearest fields were cultivated; the more distant ones became overgrown, and were used as hunting preserves; farmland had no value, because the population had so diminished that enough grain to feed them could be grown in limited cultivated areas." Large areas of central Italy became entirely vacant. Swamps developed which rendered the area even more unhealthy due to insect-borne diseases. Hieronymus wrote that the human race had been "all but destroyed" and that the earth was returning to a state of desert and forest.

Britain's history was very clearly influenced by a medieval pandemic, the nature of which is not known. In the year 444 A.D. a terrible pestilence struck Britain, an epidemic which was greatly responsible for the historically momentous conquest of Great Britain by the Saxons In fact, the Saxon chieftans were actually called upon for assistance because the Britons could no longer resist incursions from the north because of the depletion by plague of their fighting forces. So the present character of the British people, their mores, their customs, and their architecture, was greatly determined by a plague which occurred 1500 years ago.

The Roman Empire did not fall because of the Persians, the Vandals or the Goths. Rome fell primarily because of plague. The coup d'etat of Rome was not accomplished with spears and buckets of flaming oil but with the plague of Justinian. This great plague was beautifully described by Procopius:

"At this time (540 A.D.) there started a plague .... It spread over the entire earth, and afflicted all without mercy, both sexes and of every age. It began in Egypt, at Pelusium; thence it spread to Alexandria and to the rest of Egypt; then it went to Palestine, and from there over the whole earth; in such a manner that in each place it had seasonal occurrence. It spared no habitations of men, however remote they may have been. And if, at times, it seemed as though it had spared a region for a time, it would surely appear there later, not then attacking those who had been afflicted at an earlier time; and it lasted always until it had claimed its usual number of victims. It seemed always to spread inland from the coastal regions, thence penetrating deeply into the interior.

"In the second year, in the spring, it reached Byzantium and began in the following manner: to many there appeared phantoms in human form. Those who were so encountered, were struck by a blow from the phantom, and so contracted the sickness. Others locked themselves into their houses. But then the phantom appeared to them in dreams or they heard voices that told them that they had been selected for death."

Procopius, an intelligent man, reflects in this letter the utter terror, hopelessness, helplessness and panic which

27

was caused by this great pestilence. He made the interesting observation that few died at first; and then there were as many as *10,000 deaths a day*. This is a pertinent point about epidemics, their starting out slowly and appearing not to kill many people. The number of dying and dead rises with appalling violence as the pestilence gathers velocity. Our present AIDS epidemic appears to be taking a similar course.

Procopius said, "Finally, when there was a scarcity of grave diggers, the roofs were taken off the towers of the forts, the interiors filled with corpses, and the roofs replaced. Corpses were placed on ships and these abandoned to the sea. And after the plague had ceased, there was so much depravity and general licentiousness, that it seemed as though the disease had left only the most wicked."

The Roman Empire was thrown into utter confusion. The great historian Gibbon, speaking of the plague, said: "No facts have been preserved to sustain an account or even a conjecture of the numbers that perished in this extraordinary mortality. I only find, that in three months, five and ten thousand persons died each day at Constantinople; and many cities in the far east were left vacant, and that in several districts of Italy the harvest and the vintage withered on the ground. The triple scourges of war, pestilence and famine afflicted the subjects of Justinian, and his reign was disgraced by visible decrease of the human species, which has never been regained in some of the fairest countries of the globe."

The Emperor Justinian was making a mighty effort to restore the Roman Empire. The Empire was beset on all sides by Persians, Vandals and Goths. From everywhere the ring of defense was being pushed in by ever increasing hordes of barbarians. And superimposed on this was the coup d'etat of Rome—the killing, terrifying and disorganizing pestilential plague. Thus the power, the beauty, the administrative intelligence and logic of the Roman Empire died.

Before the Roman Empire, the Greeks encountered the same dreadful enemy. But in this case it was reversed and the plague was a friend of Greece rather than the destroyer. Heroditus tells us that Xerxes entered Thessalie with a gigantic army of 800,000 men. Soon after they entered disease struck, and men began to die by the thousands. Although the war appeared to be won, the campaign was abandoned and the Persian king was sent packing back to Asia—conquered by disease.

But the Athenians themselves did not fair well in the time of Pericles. A plague struck killing 65,000 men and slaves in just one year. Pericles himself succumbed to the plague. Many slaves were set free to roam across the Greek empire.

The crusaders were also defeated, not by spear, but by disease. In the year 1098 the Christian army of 300,000 men attacked the Saracen city of Antioch. Disease killed so many men in such a short period of time that the dead could not be buried. Seven thousand of their horses died of infection, but in spite of these terrible losses the city of Antioch was captured. However, on the march to Jerusalem the invisible enemy was tracking the heels of the crusaders. By the time Jerusalem was taken the original force of 300,000 men had melted down to 20,000, mostly killed by pestilence.

The second crusade, led by Louis VII of France, had an even worse experience. Of 500,000 men who started the campaign only a few managed to straggle back to Antioch, and very few of those returned to Europe. The rest died from some form of pestilence—cholera, smallpox, the black death, or typhus.

The fourth crusade under the Doge of Venice never even reached Jerusalem because of a horrible bubonic plague outbreak which totally decimated the army.

In the sixteenth century Charles V attacked the city of Metz, but again pestilence ruled the day, and the army retreated after losing 30,000 men to disease.

Emperor Maximillian II experienced the same fate. He met the sultan, Suleiman I, in Hungary. Typhus struck, and 80,000 troops were so diseased and demoralized that Maximillian retreated in disarray.

In 1632 both armies in a campaign were defeated by typhus even before they were able to join in battle. Gustavus Adolphus and Wallenstein faced each other before Nurenburg. The typhus attack quickly killed 18,000 soldiers on both sides, and both armies quickly retreated in panic.

In 1741 the city of Prague surrendered to the French army, because 30,000 Austrian soldiers had died of typhus.

The French encountered disaster in Haiti in 1801. General LeClerc was sent to Haiti with 25,000 men by Napoleon to put down a revolt. By the time the smoke had cleared 22,000 of 25,000 Frenchmen had died of yellow fever.

Even Napoleon could not win over the unseen enemy. Napoleon was defeated by typhus, not Trafalgar. After Napoleon's retreat from Moscow, which resulted primarily from pestilence, 40,000 men died from typhus. Napoleon's second army in 1813, a total of 500,000 men, was almost completely wiped out by pestilence.

The influence of great disease pandemics on military conquests throughout history has not been overlooked by our enemies.

Plague and the AIDS Epidemic

My medical dictionary gives the definition of plague as "a pestilence or severe epidemic." But an organism called Yersinia pestis has, because of its illustrious history, captured the name of plague. It is important that we understand *Y. pestis* because, not only is it the "prince of plagues," but its history can give us interesting lessons which we may need in the near future.

Another reason for studying this awesome disease is because it is always nearby, ready to pounce upon unsuspecting man yet again. Most Americans would be shocked to learn that plague-infected animals infest at least 40 percent of the continental United States. The number of cases of plague appearing in the United States is going up almost yearly. In 1983 there were 40 recorded cases.

After the biblical plague of the Philistines, the next clearly defined epidemic came in the time of Emperor Justinian around 500 A.D. Justinian's able and articulate secretary, Procopius, reported: "The bodies of the sick were covered with black pustules or carbuncles, the symptoms of immediate death .... Those who were without friends or servants lay unburied in the streets or in their desolate houses .... Corpses were placed aboard ships, and these were abandoned to the seas .... Physicians could not tell which cases were light and which severe, and no remedies availed." This pathetic and depressing description was repeated many times over the next 1500 years. At one time during the "plague of Justinian" there were 10,000 deaths per day at Constantinople.[4]

The second great plague epidemic came 600 years later and was known as the Black Death. In L347 the Crimean port of Kaffa was besieged by the Kipchak Khan. The siege went on for years, but finally an unseen warrior came to the aid of the Crimeans. Dr. Charles T. Gregg describes in eloquent detail the defeat of the Khan by this unseen enemy

---

4 Edward Gibbon, **The Decline and Fall of the Roman Empire.**

31

"In crowded and unsanitary encampments, the long imbed warriors of the Khan fell to the plague, mowed down as grass before the scythe. Furious and fearful, the Khan prepared to decamp, but before doing so, he ordered that plague-infested corpses be catapulted over the walls of Kaffa, so that he might share the pestilence with his enemy. The siege was ended as the remnants of the Khan's stricken army hurried away from their unburied dead. The Genoese traders (who had been trapped in the town) quickly sailed for their homeland. The great galleys wenched up their anchors, loosed sails from the yardarms, and bore off to the western seas bearing cargoes of jewels, nutmeg, rich cloth—and the Black Death."

So the Italian traders brought the plague to Europe. Boccaccio in the **Decameron** sounded very much like Procopius of 800 years before: "These ... maladies seemed to set entirely at naught both the art of the physician and the virtues of the physic, indeed, whether it was that the &order was of a nature to defy such treatment, or that the physicians were at fault . . . almost all died. There was now such a multitude both of men and women who practiced without having received the slightest tincture of medical science, and being in ignorance of its true causes, failed to apply the proper remedies."

There were of course no effective remedies and would not be for another 600 years. The ignorant knew as much about the Black Death as the learned, and the cure rate of those unlettered healers, the barefoot doctors, was as high as among those appropriately "tinctured" with medical education.

The plaintive wails of history are almost endless: "Father abandoned child; wife, husband; one brother, another .... And so they died. No one can be found to bury the dead for money or for friendship . . . and I, Agnola di

Tura, called the Fat, buried my five children with my own hands, and so did many others likewise."[5]

The citizens of Paris watched with dread, knowing full well that they would be next in line for this terrible pestilence. Philip VI ordered the medical faculty at the University of Paris to determine the cause of this dread disease. The learned professors, of course, had little trouble finding an etiology—it was astrology. A conjunction of Saturn, Mars and Jupiter in the house of Aquarius had caused the whole thing. Obviously, the conjunction of all three of these planets could only presage a catastrophic event.

Some skeptics pointed out that it would seem unlikely that this conjunction of planets would cause an epidemic that occurred three years later. But then, as Moliere said to the father of a recalcitrant patient, "Sir, it is better to die according to the rules than to live in contradiction to the faculty of medicine."[6] The learned doctors said that in order to avoid the disease one should avoid fatty meat. One should not sleep beyond sunrise. One should not take too many baths. And sexual intercourse could possibly be fatal.

In 1664 the plague struck London. The president of the College of Physicians and all his colleagues quickly fled the city and the Royal Society of Medicine suspended its meetings. The king, Charles II, quickly followed suit.

Dr. Nathaniel Hodges echoes Procopius and Boccaccio in his thoughts on plague: "Many patients were lost when they were thought in a safe recovery; and when we thought the conquest quite contained, death ran away with the victory; whereas others got over it, when quite given up for lost, much to the dis-refutation of our art."

The pestilence in London was so fearful in September of 1665 that in one five week period more than 38,000 Londoners were killed. As Dr. Hodges wrote, "Who

---

5 Cronica Senese.
6 L'Amour Medecin.

33

would not melt with grief to see the stock for a future generation hang upon the breasts of their dead mother? Or the marriage bed changed the first night into a sepulcher, and the unhappy pair meet with death in their first embraces."

The third great pandemic of plague, for some reason unremembered by most of the world, started about 1850. This great plague killed, in a few months, *13 million people.*

As Americans and others in the free world face the AIDS attack on their immune systems, various plagues stand by, ready to decimate modern man. The plague bacillus is now showing an increased resistance to antibiotics. This raises the terrible spectre of our most important defense, antibiotics, evaporating at the moment when it may be most needed.

Boccaccio in his great work **The Decameron** (1353) perhaps best described the mood of terror and hopelessness during the great plague: ". . . Rather it was come to this, that a dead man was then of no more account than a dead goat would be today."

The young America of the nineteenth century didn't think of plague. The Prince of Plague, Y. Pestis, was only something you read about in the history books and in the newspapers concerning faraway places like Calcutta and Istanbul. But the Prince had friends, and America was not to be immune from the devastation of plague epidemics.

A hundred years after the great yellow fever plague of Philadelphia *Yersinia pestis,* the plague after which the other plagues are all named, discovered America.

On June 28, 1899, two Oriental corpses wearing life preservers washed up on the shores of San Francisco Bay. They were both completely saturated with plague and had been in quarantine on a ship, but had jumped overboard to escape quarantine. Nine months later America had its first bubonic plague epidemic.

On March 6, 1900, a Chinese man was carried from the Globe Hotel in Chinatown, and as the death was unattended, an autopsy was required. The physician performing the autopsy noted great swollen areas in the Oriental man's groin and reported that he suspected plague. A physician for the San Francisco board of health did indeed find organisms resembling plague.

Appropriately, this was the Chinese year of the rat, and the first great plague had begun in the United States of America. It would turn out to be a very disgraceful period in the history of public health in the United States.

Things started off well enough. Chinatown was cordoned off for 12 blocks, and a search was begun for more plague cases among the 25,000 inhabitants of this rodentinfested area. The Surgeon General was called and warned that there was probably a plague epidemic in the making in the San Francisco area. Although the public health authorities at this point had been doing a creditable job, they were immediately attacked by business interests and the press in the San Francisco area. Dr. J. J. Kinyoun of the health department was ridiculed in bad verse:

Have you heard of the deadly bacillus,
Scourge of a populous land,
Bacillus that threatens to kill us,
When found in a Chinaman 's gland?

Guinea pigs were inoculated with blood from the dead Oriental. Plague organisms were recovered from these animals, confirming Koch's postulates and thus proving the presence of the plague.

However, political pressure was so great that in spite of this incontrovertible evidence of plague, the quarantine was lifted in Chinatown in only 60 hours. To their discredit, the Pacific Medical and Surgical Journal supported the business interests in deriding the evidence of plague.

But no credit is due to the Chinese of the area; they also refused to cooperate and hid dead Chinese from inspectors. The Board of Supervisors of San Francisco apparently began to grasp the seriousness of the situation and established a cordon around Chinatown. The California Board of Health asked for the help of the governor, Mr. Henry T. Gage. Gage refused to cooperate in any way with the San Francisco authorities. He even ordered that the quarantine of Chinatown be terminated.

Gage made "an investigation" and then concluded that "plague did not nor ever did exist in California." He then proceeded to fire the members of the state Board of Health, including the state bacteriologist who originally uncovered the epidemic. By June of the next year there had been 61 confirmed deaths in San Francisco from plague; undoubtedly there were many, many more unconfirmed cases, yet the governor remained adamant.

The governor, although he had already made a complete ass of himself, made the incredible allegation that the plague bacillus had actually been isolated by the health authorities from imported cultures. He went on to say that a bill should be passed that would make transportation of plague cultures without his permission a crime punishable by life imprisonment. It would be a felony to broadcast the presence of plague in San Francisco!

By this time, to their eternal credit, the Board of Health and much of California's medical profession now recognized the clear danger that they faced and were demanding action against the plague. The Chinese community, railroad and shipping interests, newspapers and merchants associations still, along with the newly constituted Board of Health, declared that plague did not exist in California, never did and never would. Finally, in spite of help from the governor and his ignorant and fanatical business friends, the plague went away. The total death count was 122 with *an apparent mortality rate of 97 percent.*

Because rabbits are the most common source of plague in the United States, the condition is often mis-diagnosed as tuleremia, a common infection of rabbits which can be transmitted to man. The mis-diagnosis is important because the treatments for tularemia and plague infection are different. This mistake can be crucial with a concurrent AIDS infection—leading to fulminating plague disease and death.

Another common mm-diagnosis is inguinal hernia. The doctor sees a swelling in the groin and assumes it is an entrapped piece of intestine causing a hernia. It will be swollen and sore, and the two are extremely difficult to tell apart. If the doctor is not accustomed to seeing plague he will diagnose it as an incarcerated inguinal hernia every time. Because of the swelling of a venereal disease called granuloma inguinalli or lymphogranuloma venerum may also be mis-diagnosed as an inguinal hernia. Also mononucleosis and any other infection that causes the swelling of the lymph nodes can mislead the physician. You can imagine the surgeon's surprise when he takes the patient to surgery and starts to operate on an "inguinal hernia," and when his knife enters the swelling a gigantic spurt of pus greets him between the eyes.

The pneumonic, or respiratory form of plague is almost always mis-diagnosed as "pneumonia." Often before the proper diagnosis of pneumonic plague is made the patient is beyond help and will die even if the appropriate antibiotics, streptomycin and chloromycetin, are given in massive doses.

It is not difficult to imagine the chaos and terror that would come with the rapid spread of plague during the AIDS epidemic. With the weakened immune system caused by AIDS, the infection with plague is almost certain to be fatal in almost every case even if a proper and timely treatment is given.

A classical example of the difficulty in diagnosing and treating plague, even under normal circumstances without the AIDS epidemic, is illustrated by the study of 38 plague cases in children in New Mexico between 1979 and 1980.

Only eight percent of the children were initially suspected of having plague at the time of their hospitalization, even though New Mexico is the most common plague state in the United States. They were undiagnosed even though 82 percent of these children had typical, classical buboes in their groins.

The average time from onset of the illness to death was just over four days. Of the six fatal cases, four *never* received an effective antibiotic treatment; two received treatment at the day of death. There was an average delay of *nearly four days f*rom the onset of illness until effective treatment was prescribed. Young lives are lost every year because of the average physician's inability to make a prompt and accurate diagnosis and then follow it up with effective antibiotic therapy.

Modern and rapid transportation has compounded this problem of diagnosis and treatment of plague. A plague victim can, before his symptoms appear, hop on an airplane in Albuquerque, New Mexico, and turn up with full blown plague disease in places as remote from the plague center as Greenville, South Carolina. This did indeed happen when Donna Delattre contracted plague from a wild chipmunk in Santa Fe, New Mexico. Donna, after handling a dying chipmunk, left the next day and flew to Atlanta, and then was driven to Seneca, South Carolina. Because of the alert thinking of the local physician, plague was considered as she was a recent arrival from New Mexico. Donna was transferred to a large regional medical center in Greenville, South Carolina, but, despite adequate treatment with intravenous chloromycetin, she died soon after admission.

This type of "travelers' plague" is an ever increasing problem and one that is certain to bring plague to AIDS victims. "Travelers' plague" has resulted in cases of bubonic plague being reported in Texas, Massachusetts, Nebraska, South Carolina and New Orleans.

It is only a matter of time before plague will be reported in AIDS cases, because unfortunately, the rat flea xenopsylla cheopis has become resistant to DDT and rats have become resistant to warfarin, the rat poison that has worked so well in the past. With warfarin-resistant rats and DDT-resistant fleas we are back to square-one in plague control, i.e., we're back to 1930. Our only resistance to this fearful disease is the antibiotics streptomycin and chloromycetin. Both of these are in minimum supply at most treatment areas, and it is highly unlikely that most hospitals would have enough available to give effective treatment during an epidemic.

To illustrate the ubiquitousness of the plague organism, and why man must remain constantly alert to this devastating disease, a septacemia case is reported from Colorado Springs, Colorado. A 11month-old girl died from septacemic plague on September 3, 1984. She was the daughter of an Air Force officer *and her home was on the Air Force Academy grounds!* The source of the infection was unknown, possibly from a pet cat.

From there we jump a third of the way around the world to Saudi Arabia where, in 1984, nine people caught bubonic plague from an infected camel after he was butchered and eaten. The two butchers and seven members of his family died.

It is truly remarkable how the ancient wisdom of centuries is ignored by contemporary doctors. In the last years of the nineteenth century there were vicious plagues in both Hong Kong and India, but the British authorities mis-read the situation. As Shih Tao-nan had pointed out a hundred years before, the dying of rats presaged the beginning of an epidemic of plague in humans. But the British doctors with this information right

39

under their noses claimed that the rats caught the plague from the humans! As the rats die the infected fleas leave the carcasses of the rats and go to man, thus giving humans the plague. One wonders with our present dreadful plague epidemic how many "obvious" things of this nature are keeping us from the truth of the epidemiology of AIDS. Right or wrong the medical authorities are always very definite and positive about their opinions. The British-Indian plague commission in 1899 reported, "There is absolutely *no evidence* that the disease has ever been carried from one country to another by plague-infected rats and ships." The editor of the Indian Medical Gazette said in 1902 that the rat/flea/human mode of transmission theory had been "completely demolished" and was "worthless." Medical authorities tell us today that AIDS simply cannot be transmitted by mosquitoes— "ridiculous," "unscientific."

Will history repeat?

The plague's lieutenants–rats and fleas–are standing by in the countryside waiting for immune systems of Americans to become so depleted that they can move in for the kill. Plague is endemic in almost all of the western states with many animals, including rats, rabbits, squirrels, prairie dogs and others being infested by plague-infected fleas.

Rats are everywhere, and it is said that there is one rat for every person in the city of New York.

Robert Browning described man's frustration with the rat:

Rats!
They fought the dogs and killed the cats,
And bit the babies in the cradles,
And ate the cheeses out of the vats,
And licked the soup from the cook's own ladles.[7]

---

7 7he Pied Piper of Hamlin, 1845.

The rat is a truly formidable enemy with which we may have a life and death struggle in the near future. The rat is one of the few animals, which of course includes man, that kills for pleasure. The rats' incisor teeth grow five inches a year, and so they are gnawing incessantly. They can penetrate concrete, lead pipes and cinder block. They will also eat plastic, aluminum, fiberboard and asbestos. He can enter a hole hardly larger than the diameter of an adult human forefinger. They are a truly destructive, prolific and murderous enemy.

The New York estimate may be low. In Akron, Ohio, for instance, there was found to be about 25 rats per person; and in Texarkana they found 15 rats per human. The rat has an unwanted traveler in the flea, known as Xenopsylla Cheopis.

Although AIDS is indeed a deadly peril, the pneumonic form of plague is an even more infectious and deadly disease, perhaps being exceeded in ferocity only by botulism. If an enemy were to attack us with pneumonic plague and we were in a debilitated condition due to the weakening of our immune systems through AIDS and AIDS-like diseases, the devastation would be total. The pneumonic plague is uniformly fatal unless treated within hours of the appearance of symptoms. This would be highly unlikely for 99 percent of the population during an emergency. If this were to occur, the only people to survive would be those lucky enough not to have an AIDS-induced weakening of the immune system. Even those might not survive a *pneumonic* plague epidemic. By comparison, the simple bubonic plague is a "benign" disease. About 25-50 percent of the victims of bubonic plague recover without treatment.

We face a new "designer gene" technology in which a germ can be engineered which will have a built in resistance to antibiotics. But with a pneumonic plague epidemic this would not be necessary because few hospitals would have adequate supplies of the antibiotics required for curing early pneumonic plague.

The frustration and utter hopelessness that man, including Americans, have felt concerning plague was well described in a paragraph from Dr. Charles T. Gregg's book **Plague**:

"Each member of the plague trinity (rat/flea/*yersinia pestis* microbe) is tough, adaptable and prolific. Together they constitute a formidable force, undeterred in the path by man's puny efforts to turn it aside. Plague has worn seven-league boots, a cloak of invincibility, and an air of disdain. Nothing man has done against it ever mattered very much. Humanitys lot was to weep with rage, frustration and fear as plague swept to and fro unheeded. Bonfires in the streets, pograms, amulets, magic potion or solemn Mass, together or separately, had no effect. Plague struck with demented fury, turned away, then struck again, as if mocking man's impotence."

A grimly funny example of frustration was the effort to eliminate rats in order to eliminate plague during the European pestilence. Rat poisons have always been sold with the idea that they will cause the rat to leave the house before he dies. This is essential to avoid the stench of dead rats and the escape of the plague-carrying fleas from rats to humans. A poem was written about the mythical rat killer called "Tuff-on Rats":

Johnny and the other brats,
Ate up all the 'Tuff-on Rats'
Father said, as Mother cried,
'Never mind, they'll die outside.'

In view of the AIDS epidemic the plague spectre looms ever larger. Dr. M. Baltazard said in 1960, "The silence of plague today must not blind us to the fact that its present positions are stronger than ever before; entrenched within reach of all the strongholds of modern civilization, it may well be a disease of the future."

In studying the long cyclic swings of history and pestilence one realizes that judgment of political, cultural, sexual and other changes in human behavior and destinies must be based on a period of two or three hundred years. With our own limited experience we can apprize only a fraction of the curve in the cycle of which we are a part, and we cannot look forward clearly unless we are trained and capable of looking back to the beginning of our particular historical curve.

Stanford University, Palo Alto, California, (A "Fictionized" True Story)

Tony Neel peered into his microscope. He was looking at *Xenopsylla cheopis*, the oriental rat flea, which carries the plague.

Neel had always been fascinated by this amazing creature which had played such a significant part in the history of war for thousands of years. He called it the "fabulous flea": wingless, flattened and equipped at one end with a very efficient syringe- for sucking blood and on the other with a propulsion system that, compared to the size of man, enables it to jump the equivalent of a sixty story building. Cheopis can leap clear across the average room. He can walk straight up a vertical sheet of glass some 20,000 times his own length. The magnificent cheetah and the graceful dolphin are mere slugs compared to the fabulous flea.

Fleas are from the family Siphonaptera, meaning a wingless siphon, and siphon they do with great efficiency. In a few minutes they suck up their own weight in blood. If you weigh 150 pounds, can you imagine taking in 150 pounds of food in two minutes?

Tony Neel was a flea specialist and he got a lot of kidding about it: "carrying his pets in a matchbox," "Hide

43

your dog, here comes Tony" and the like. But Neel's scientific mission was deadly serious, the search for Yersinia pestis, the organism that fleas carry to humans, thus causing bubonic plague, the Black Death.

Neel had found the plague organism in fleas captured from rats in San Francisco and south to San Bruno Mountain which is half way from fashionable Nob Hill to the San Francisco International Airport. Today was to bring a disturbing revelation. The fleas under his microscope were taken from the Stanford University campus. They were loaded with the plague bacillus!

Neel knew what most San Francisco area residents did not: San Francisco had had two plague epidemics in the first 10 years of the twentieth century. He also knew that the plague flea, *X. cheopis*, was waiting patiently on the backs of millions of rats for a breakdown in sanitation to again attack man with the Black Death.

He thought with apprehension about the recent announcement by doctors in San Francisco, less than an hour away from Stanford, that they feared a complete breakdown in health services because of the crushing burden of thousands of dying AIDS patients. A "breakdown in health services" meant far more than the man in the street realized, he mused. Sanitation would deteriorate and the plague would move in.

RECOMMENDED READING:

McNeill, **Plagues and Peoples,** Doubleday-Anchor Books, Garden City, New York, 1976.

Zinsser, **Rats, Lice and History,** Little, Brown & Co., Boston, 1963.

Gregg, **Plague**, Univ. Mexico Press, Albuquerque, 1985.
Gottfried, The Black Death, Free Press, N.Y.

Chapter 2
The Future of AIDS

People give little thought to how delicate the social fabric really is. A major assault on this delicate balance, such as AIDS, affects everyone. If 10 million are sick and dying it will take 50 million of the worried well to take care of them. Many people are already refusing to take care of AIDS patients. When St. Vincent's Hospital of New York went to Britain to recruit operating room nurses it had no takers for fear of AIDS. Who is going to take care of these dying and suffering people?

It will be impossible to take care of them. There would be no one left to run the country. AIDS death houses will develop where a tacit euthanasia and even de facto murder will be practiced. Crematories will work around the clock. With massive dying, such as occurred in Germany in 1944 and 1945, mostly due to starvation, typhus and cholera, mass graves and cremation are the only way to protect the living from even more pestilence and infection.

Do you consider the above scenario to be preposterous in a modern country? Listen to an expert, Mindell Seidlin, director of the Bellevue AIDS program: "The medicines they receive are big guns with a lot of side-effects and toxicity. They have many diagnostic procedures. They are weak, debilitated, can't feed themselves, they need help to the bathroom and have severe diarrhea. *And 30 percent develop dementia.*" (Emphasis added.) It is now believed that all AIDS-infected persons have moderate to severe mental impairment and most will develop dementia, especially children with AIDS.

Eventually, because of shortages, antibiotics will be withheld from AIDS patients. There will be protests (at first) of discrimination. But what do you do if half the people in a life boat are obviously dying and the boat is sinking because of overload? There is no doubt in my mind that AIDS patients will be abandoned in AIDS death houses to take care of each other until death do them part. They will die of an unimaginable garden variety of terrible diseases including starvation, tubercu10sis, syphilis, pneumocystis pneumonia, torula meningitis, plague, Kaposi's sarcoma cancer (which virtually rots the body away inside and out), leukemia, yeast septicemia, suicide and murder.

During the first great plague, physicians fled from the centers of pestilence just like everyone else. The great physician, Galen, put it bluntly: "Flee the plague and live to treat another day." And that's exactly what he did. A surgeon in Wisconsin has refused to perform heart surgery on AIDS-infected persons. This rejection will spread as more health care workers refuse to risk their lives for a person doomed to die.

The ancient physician, Rhazes, was more poetic than Galen:

"Three little words the plague dispel"
quick, far; and late, where 'ere you dwell
Start quick go far and right away,
and your return till late delay."

Two and a half percent of pregnant women at King's County Hospital in New York are now positive for AIDS. AIDS has increased five-fold in two years in straight-laced Switzerland' They have an estimated 20,000 carriers.[1] A burn victim in England has caught AIDS from a skin graft.[2] According to the Centers for Disease Control, an American woman has contracted AIDS from a bone

---

1 *Am. Med. News*, 2/13/87.

2 Op. Cit., 3/13187.

graft.[3] Twenty-eight patients worldwide have become infected through transplants or artificial insemination.[4]

The Haitian experience portends what will happen here. In 1983, 71 percent of AIDS cases were among homosexuals and 29 percent were among heterosexuals. In only two years the trend completely reversed itself with 11 percent homosexual and 70 percent heterosexual. Ominous.

The National Institute of Health has announced that an AIDS researcher has been infected with the virus.[5] He always wore gloves when handling the virus. This NIH report gave out some disinformation concerning AIDS. They said that this is "the first known instance of the virus being contracted in a laboratory setting." Eight laboratory workers at the Pasteur Institute in Paris are dead or dying of AIDS or an AIDS-like virus, probably HTLV-I or an SV-40 recombinant.

Over five percent of all AIDS-infected people work in hospitals.[6] Ian Carr, M.D., Cook County Hospital, says "causal contact is one way you can't get AIDS." Does "casual contact" include sticking a needle in your arm, putting a catheter in your bladder, and poking a tube down your throat? Even if Carr were right, he's wrong because: *AIDS-infected people tend to carry other high) infectious diseases* such as a virulent form of tuberculosis, a deadly hepatitis and torula histolytica, a uniformly fatal type of meningitis.

The Surgeon General and the politicians are endangering all of us through their refusal to face the reality of this devastating plague and the other diseases it brings with it.

---

3 *Atlanta Journal and Constitution*, 10/7/88.
4 Ibid.
5 *Associated Press*, September 12,1987.
6 *Newsweek*, 9/24/87.

If the experts think that you can't get AIDS from casual contact, then why are hospitals trying to get rid of employees who have AIDS? Do they know something we don't? AIDS-related job discrimination is skyrocketing.[7]

The CDC says it's perfectly safe for AIDS-infected persons to work in hospitals as long as they follow the " 1985 barrier guidelines." Do you believe that irresponsible people who flaunt all social and sexual mores will follow CDC guidelines?

An interesting quote from the Wall Street Journal: "Some say that it is only a matter of time before the most important occupations at Eighth and M Streets (Washington, DC)—prostitution and drug dealing—are supplanted by the work of undertakers."[8]

Blue Cross is worried about going broke, especially in California. One official stated that "we are deeply worried" and that the cost for claims will be into the billions by the mid-90's. "By 1995 we could be paying more for treatment of AIDS than we pay out today for all health care claims."

Some state legislatures are now forcing the insurance companies to insure applicants even if they have a positive blood test for AIDS. This will bankrupt the insurance industry ($200,000 per case) and totally state-controlled medicine will quickly follow.

Dr. James Curran of the CDC, who has not been exactly a paragon of honesty concerning AIDS prevention, is finally starting to panic, He said at a February, 1988 AIDS meeting in Atlanta that AIDS infection is at least 50 times larger than the 31,000 recorded cases. Let's see now. Fifty times 31,000 is 1.5 million plus another 50,000.

Each of the four international conferences on AIDS has had its own particular character. The first one in

---

7 *Am. Med. News*, 2/27/87
8 *Wall Street Journal*, 11/4/87.

Atlanta, Georgia, in 1985, was delivered with a sense *of shock*.

The second one in Paris was with an atmosphere *full of gloom*.

The 1987 conference in Washington was characterized by "restraint with real optimism."[9]

The 1988 meeting in Stockholm reflected a mood of *despair*:

Misinformation on AIDS continues to come from the media, even in reliable publications such as the British publication, *New Scientist*. *New Scientist* says: "AIDS spreads most rapidly where education is poor, social conditions are miserable and health services are inadequate."

This is a gross oversimplification and an inadequate description of how AIDS actually spreads. AIDS in Africa, for instance, started in the cities among the upper middle class of the various equatorial states. AIDS in the United States started among the upper socio-economic homosexual group in New York, Los Angeles and San Francisco. It only became a disease of the poverty class when the epidemic broke out into intravenous drug users. As AIDS is spread most efficiently through needles, it only took a few homosexuals in the IV drug culture to cause it to spread like wildfire through that subculture.

Dr. Otis R. Bowen of Health and Human Services, is more candid than many: "We face the dreadful prospect of a worldwide death toll in the tens of millions a decade from now." He predicts a possible 100 million within 20 years. Bowen doesn't pull any punches. He describes the "awesome proportions of the worst health problem in the history of the world."

Dr. Stanley Monteith of Santa Cruz, California said the "AIDS epidemic will destroy the very fabric of this nation within the next few years if immediate public health

---

9 *New Scientist*, 6/23/88.

measures are not taken to bring this plague under control. I only hope and pray it is already not too late. If AIDS simply doubles eight more times within the next 10 years about 10 million people will be dead and dying and ten times that many will carry the virus. That will spell the end of the American dream."[10]

Dr. James Mason, director of the CDC, said that he would recommend "strong legislation to prevent discrimination against carriers of the virus." So the person who mixes your I.V. at the hospital, your dentist or the doctor who operates on you may harbor the AIDS virus, *but you have no right to know.*

Dr. James W. Curran, director of AIDS research at the Centers for Disease Control, was interviewed recently by American Medical News (VlSl8B). While Mason, his boss, worries about &crimination, Dr. Curran reported:

- *For the U.S. the outlook it very sobering* and we must conclude that AIDS is endemic to the U.S. (Endemic means it's here to stay).
- During the last 12 months there have been 20,000 *new cases of AIDS.*
- Ninety percent will die within three years of diagnosis.
- We are looking at *hundreds of thousands* of AIDS patients who in the near future will require lifetime care.
- The risk to heterosexuals remains unknown.
- The leading AIDS states *per capita:*
  1) Washington, D.C.
  2) New York
  3) California
  4) New Jersey

10 *AAM News,* 1/15/88.

5) Florida
6) Texas
7) Maryland
8) Hawaii
9) Connecticut
10) Massachusetts tied with Georgia

- A vaccine for AIDS is the "longest shot." (See Chapter 9.)
- The epidemic has not plateaued.

Did you know that all full-blown AIDS patients, no matter what their age, are rewarded with Social Security Disability? Soon the debate as to whether Social Security is bankrupt will end. There will be no Social Security.

If we can't quarantine AIDS-positive people then we should at least punish the ones who are irresponsible. Anyone who knows he has AIDS and who infects another should be prosecuted for second degree murder. Conviction should mean a mandatory life sentence.

Like cancer, there will be a lot more money made in "treating" rather than curing AIDS. The AMA is going down the same old drug trail it went down with cancer. The result will be the same: the squandering of millions of dollars on useless and toxic "chemo-therapeutic" drugs. As with cancer it's really chemo-euthanasia.

The *AMA News* of November 7, 1986, headlined a report on AZT: "AZT Success, Despite Side Effects." They showed a picture, next to the heading, of a young, healthy looking AIDS patient. He reports exuberantly, "If I didn't know I was sick, I wouldn't know I was sick." The implication is that AZT is working. It does *not* work and most patients discontinue it because of the devastating side effects. How can a drug that weakens the immune system be good for an immune deficiency?

Keep in mind that the very scientists who were supposed to deliver us from cancer through Nixon's "War on

Cancer" are the same scientists who are supposed to deliver us from the AIDS epidemic.

"Three decades of medical research have failed to stop the rising rate of death from cancer among Americans " reports Michael Waldholz in the *Wall Street Journal*.[11] "Despite the optimistic pronouncements of many federal Officials and cancer specialists," Waldholz said, "true respected public health researchers charge in the report that 'we are losing the war against cancer.' " In the past 20 years cancer deaths have risen 8.7 percent.

Bio-statistician John C. Bailar III from Harvard University School of Public Health said, "The bottom line is that despite all the billions of dollars, the promises, and the claims of success, more people are dying of cancer than before, and to say otherwise is to mislead the American people into believing we are beating this problem."

John Cairns, also of the Harvard School of Public Health said, "But any impression that we are on the verge of defeating the disease is wrong, and the opposite may well be true."

In a very real sense, cancer is AIDS and AIDS is cancer. A deficient immune system is the very basis for all disease, whether inherited or contracted. The reason you die of cancer is because your immune system cannot combat the virus. The reason one dies of AIDS is also because one enact combat this viral disease. The only distinction between cancer of the past and cancer of the present is that now we have highly infectious forms of cancer. The same people are fighting the same old battle in the same old ways. If these scientists upon whom we are depending for a cure do not free their minds up and consider new approaches, such as electromagnetic and vibrational medicine, there is little hope for our survival.

---

11 5/8/86.

Now For the Really Bad News

Dr. Robert Redfield of Walter Reed Army Medical Center predicts that 10 million Americans may be infected by 1991. But statistical expert Donald E. Babcock, Ph.D., says these figures are grossly inaccurate. Using the official data, he predicts 23 million deaths within two years, 1991. The number infected but still alive could be 10 times as much or 230 million—meaning everybody. As all AIDS positive individuals will eventually die, probably within 10 years, modern civilization and possibly the human race could disappear within two decades.

Preposterous? British expert Dr. John Seale has stated that the AIDS virus might "render the human race extinct within 50 years"[12] He is optimistic. Anthropologists have wondered how civilizations, like the Incas, just disappeared. Was it a retroviral plague?

Dr. Babcock, an able writer as well as able statistician, said he analyzed the AIDS situation "to determine what the import was of what we were being told by the numerous authorities, clairvoyants and soothsayers about the facts, near-facts and blatant fictions about the AIDS plague now upon us.

---

12 *The New American,* Jan. 19,1987.

Dr. Babcock said, "Knowing that the U.S. Government by international treaty was involved in the 'Global 2000' policy of being a participant in the possible eradication of a billion or more people from the face of this earth by the year 2000 using whatever method was required, whether they be wars, disease, starvation, plagues or whatever, I was not surprised at the facts that have been given to us nor the fictions either.

"Since no other plague has been experienced that has this disease pathology or death-dealing mechanism which we face in this instance, the probability is that if no decline becomes apparent in the fatality rate rather soon the prognostications look rather bleak from any serological point of view. Some decline in the rate of propagation must of necessity occur as the disease infects a wider range of the populace. It can absolutely not be a natural wonder created by any evolutionary change. It must have had the help of a human mind gone off its moral rocker.

"If this disease was developed by human ingenuity we have out done ourselves this time, and it is to be hoped that those minds and lives that created this monster have already been destroyed by it and are now resting uncomfortably in Lucifer's hottest Wok Pot.

"Fear is the only protection available to the ignorant, or uneducated or uninformed. It is the lack of fear that kills off those who ought to know better.

"Telling us there is an induction period of from one to several years in this disease is only to tell us that the future is far more bleak than we believed before; *it only makes the probability of human obliteration more certain.*"

"In any event, unless the data change their growth rates, by the end of 1991 we will have one and one half times as many living AIDS patients for every live healthy one.

"As I think back I remember that the meaning of the name America means heavenly kingdom, and it sure looks like that is where the last remnants of America will be by 1992, when I look at these tables."

Ostrich, Inc.

The business community is living in a dream world. Control Data Corporation is typical. Bob Jones, director of their health services, said, "We wouldn't have a policy on AIDS any more than we'd have a policy on heart attacks." (Stockholders please note.)

Ford Motor Company says that it has "no reason to believe" that any of its 382,000 employees has AIDS. (Sell short.)

The insurance companies aren't dumb. When the District of Columbia banned insurance companies from testing for AIDS in effect tying the AIDS can to their tail, they simply abandoned Washington. Eighty percent of the 600 insurance companies doing business there have left. The rest are sure to follow.

Bank of America rep Nancy Merritt says proudly, "We have taken a stand." That stand is to favor the AIDS-infected person over employees who refuse to expose themselves to the danger of hepatitis, tuberculosis, and AIDS. Two pregnant women refused to work with an AIDS victim. Bank of America said quit if you're going to be so "irrational," so they did. Can you imagine two pregnant women being told that they must work with an AIDS-infected person? But that's San Francisco.

You might say that *Business Week magazine* sets the tone for American companies. *Business Week* is bullish on a cure. They say "an intense research effort is making headway," and "AIDS remains unusually hard to get." They are still telling their readers that "outside the body the virus is fragile" and "it can't be spread through food or water." All of the above may be untrue.

A recent Harris poll confirms that American business, like *Business Week,* has its head planted firmly in the sand. Only 14 percent of executives polled are greatly concerned about AIDS, and only 9 percent have even considered testing prospective employees for AIDS.

One of the most startling reports on AIDS never made the papers. Dr. Robert Gallo and Dr. Flossie Wong-Staal reported that healthy AIDS-infected persons, i.e., those with no symptoms of AIDS, are more infectious than those with symptoms of AIDS. "In our experience," report Wong-Staal and Gallo, "patients with AIDS have less virus in their blood than 'healthy, carriers *and virus was isolated from saliva of healthy carriers,* not from people with AIDS."[13]

This finding has momentous implications. Should children with AIDS be allowed to mingle freely with other children because they have no symptoms of A1DS? Are they now possibly more infectious rather than less when they are without symptoms? What about an infected flight attendant in the enclosed space, and recirculated air of a jet aircraft?

In light of this finding is "confidentiality" really fair to the uninfected portion of the population? Shouldn't people have the right to make their own decision as to whether they want to risk exposure of themselves in the workplace or their children at school?

On-The-Job AIDS Underreported

Dr. Scott Croxson of New York claims that more health care workers are getting infected with the HIV virus than are being reported. Croxson, at the international AIDS meeting in Stockholm, said: "Seroconversions are occurring despite posters at this meeting declaring otherwise. I

13 *Nature,* Vol. 317, 3 Oct., 1985.

submit that these data do not completely describe the situation that is occurring in the real world."

Although the Centers for Disease Control concede that the risk to health care workers will increase,14 the CDC says there is "no cause for concern."

American business has undertaken a campaign to convince workers that they have nothing to fear from working with an AIDS-infected person. But a large proportion of the working population is not convinced.

A survey by the Georgia Tech Center for Work Performance Problems in Atlanta, Georgia, polled 2000 workers across the country to determine their attitude toward working with AIDS patients. Two-thirds of the respondents said they would be concerned about using the same bathroom as an AIDS sufferer on the job, 40 percent were concerned about using the same cafeteria and 37 percent said they would not be willing to use the same equipment as an AIDS patient.

"If a company can expect 35-40 percent of its work force to be afraid of using the cafeteria or to refuse to share equipment, that has serious implications," said David M. Herold, Professor of Management at Georgia Tech. "If people are catatonic because they have a co-worker with AIDS, the impact on productivity and efficiency is going to be great," he added.

Although "experts" have declared that you cannot catch AIDS though casual contact, 35 percent of those surveyed simply did not believe it. Also of interest, 42 percent said it was "likely" that an AIDS sufferer would hide the illness from employers and co-workers.

Thirteen health care workers at an Illinois hospital contracted tuberculosis from one single AIDS patient. The

14 *Family Practice News.* Vol. 18 #14.

variety of tuberculosis they contracted was probably *my-cobacterium avium intracellularae for which there is no effective treatment.*[15]

There have been reported to the Centers For Disease Control 152 HIV-positive (AIDS) cases in hospital workers without "readily identified" risk factors, i.e., homosexuality, drug use, etc.

Using complicated statistical methods, a "Kaplan-Meier plot," scientists from the UCLA Biostatistics department reported that "by July, 1987 the estimated total number of cases of AIDS will be approximately 51,000".[16] We now have about 57,000 cases. Their estimate was not far off. But the CDC now admits that the total number of infected people is "at least 50 times larger" than the number of reported cases. Fifty times 57,000 is 2,850,000 infected people—*and we don't even how who they are.*

People magazine was right on target about the media. A poll of the national media elite, published in *Public Opinion* magazine and reported by *People*, revealed that 76 percent believe that homosexuality is not wrong. People lambasted the television networks for their constant portrayal of casual sex. The bodies are beginning to stack up and even *People* magazine is starting to panic.

---

15 *AIDS Protection*, June, 1988.
16 *I. Inf. Dis.*, 154, #4, October, 1986.

Chapter 3
They Shoot Mad Dogs, Don't They?

The blockbuster news about the prairie fire spread of HTLV-I leukemia gives the AIE)S epidemic an entirely new dimension. We now have two deadly plagues spreading around the world simultaneously, maybe three. Five percent of the people of Jamaica are infected with HTLV-I leukemia. It is widespread in the United States and eight percent of the Japanese people on the island of Kyushu (Japan's second most populated island) are infected.

In one way you are better off with HTLV-I, Adult T-cell leukemia/lymphoma (ATL), because you will be dead in three months. But there is a down-side to this. If you contract the neurological form called tropical spastic paraparesis (TSP), you will die a long, agonizing death with a lifetime of stiffened limbs, pain and total dependency. It's very similar to multiple sclerosis, only worse.

This deadly cousin to AIDS has been found in Africa (reported there first), Latin America, the United States, Japan, Britain, New Guinea, the Seychelles, and the Caribbean. A nice distribution for a pandemic. Only now, eight years into the epidemic, are they gearing up to test the blood supply for HTLV-I.

Dr. Robert Gallo of the National Cancer Institute says that these killer cancer viruses are "the first great pandemic of the second half of the 20th century."

That statement is not quite correct. Small pox (*Variola*), the black plague (*Yersinia pestis*), and cholera (*Vibrio*) infected most areas of the world at one time or another. But this is the first time that every country in the world has been infected at the same time with a deadly disease.

Never in recorded history has man faced anything close to this kind of biological disaster.

The latest reports state that HTLV-I is not prevalent in the United States. Not prevalent? Twenty-four thousand Americans are already believed to be infected. Fifty-six percent of drug users in Jersey City, New Jersey, are now infected with HTLV-I. On a recent CBS interview with a prostitute in Miami she admitted that she had had sex with two hundred men since she had been diagnosed as having AIDS. Does she also have HTLV-I? Is it extreme to recommend the death penalty for anyone passing these diseases knowingly to someone else? They shoot mad dogs don't they?

Health officials in Jamaica are scratching their heads as to why this new black death affects mostly the poor people. No one seems to have suggested checking the mosquitos. Jamaican doctors formally petitioned the head of the Jamaican National Transfusion Service, Dr. Grace Lindo-Haynes, to screen blood for the new killer virus. She said that she would need "more evidence" which would take about a year! (Shades of CDC).

Bonnie (HTLV-I) and Clyde (AIDS) are working together to solve the population problem. Many of the infected are carrying both viruses. Speaking of the population problem, did you know that the "Global 2,000" report, a brainchild of the Carter administration, called for a reduction of the world's population to two billion by the year 2000? Do you suppose there's any connection with AIDS? (See Chapter 4.)

Clavel and his associates isolated AIDS-II in 1986 in Africa. "We may reasonably expect this virus to be circulating in the countries outside Africa,"[1] he said. It has already been reported in England.

1 Karpas, et. al., *Lancet*, 7/18/87.

Now we have AIDS III (HTLV-V) to deal with.[2] The Pasteur Institute of Paris now reports that the "African" HTLV-V virus, previously thought to be benign, is also lethal. The experts concluded from their most recent study[3] that a new epidemic is possible in West Africa. AIDS III, like AIDS-I and AIDS-II, is probably a man-made retrovirus.

In attempting to find a vaccine for AIDS prevention, scientists have come up with 10 more varieties of the AIDS virus,[4] HTLV-I, II, III, Nigerian X and many others. Scientists disagree on how virulent these new strains are. The French say they are worried. The American scientists pretend they are not.

Dr. Robert Gallo says that "There's one real AIDS epidemic. There's one real AIDS virus." Maybe. The Pasteur Institute keeps coming up with new ones.

On June 4, 1987, Dr. Anthony Fauci of the National Institute of Allergy said, "I don't believe AIDS will ever leap into the general population of the United States." But two paragraphs down in the same article Dr. James Curran of the Centers for Disease Control says that one out of every 30 American men now are infected with AIDS. In San Francisco half of the adult male population carries the virus.[5]

The public is confused about ARC (AIDS-related Complex). That's because the doctors have confused the issue. There's no such thing as ARC. ARC is early AIDS or AIDS in a person with an unusually strong immune system. One of the experts on the Nightline "Town Hall" meeting on AIDS[6] admitted: "You can die of ARC." If you can die of ARC doesn't that make it AIDS?

---

2 *New England Journal Med.*, 316:1180 -1185,1987.
3 Ibid.
4 *Medical Trib.*, 7/8/87, report on the International AIDS conference 1984, Washington, D.C
5 A.C.A.M. Conference, Nov., 1987, Las Vegas, NV.
6 ABC, 6/5/87.

A few shockers came out of the "AIDS Town Hall Meeting" with Ted Koppel in early 1988. Doctor Stephen Joseph, Health Commissioner of New York City, said: "The leading cause of death in New York City in women between the ages of 25 and 29 is now AIDS."

A correspondent from Africa reported that in the capital of Zaire 20 percent of the citizens now have the AIDS infection. Is that a portent of what we are facing in five to 10 years? No one really knows, but the African shadow looms ever larger. Now that two new and lethal strains of AIDS have been brought to Europe by African and European businessmen the situation looks extremely grim. Now we are back to a problem of testing. The present test is no good for the new menace of HTLV-I. Many strains of flu have developed—the "Asian" flu, the "swine" flu, the "Hong Kong" flu. There is a new one every year or so. Is this going to happen with the AIDS virus? Can we develop a new test every year?

Many people have fallen for the government AIDS disinformation campaign orchestrated by Surgeon General Koop: "You can't catch it through casual contact."

This constantly reiterated mantra is of course quite vague. If you ask the experts, "What if a person with AIDS sneezes in my face and that person has tuberculosis, yeast infection of the mouth, or pneumocistis pneumonia?" "Well, that might not be so good," they will reply.

People have such a pathetic trust in science and scientists that they have taken leave of their senses. Peggy and Allison of Worcester, Massachusetts, have taken into their home three baby girls with severe, terminal AIDS.[7] These children have or have had chicken pox with open sores, brain infections, skin cancers, abscess in the mouth, runny noses from nasal infections, and severe yeast infec-

---

7   *New York Times*, 9/13/87.

tions of the mouth. Yet, the *New York Times* reports, "The women kiss and cuddle the children constantly." Peggy and Allison say they take seminars on coping with death. They will need it to cope with their *own* death from AIDS.

A state adoption agency reports that they have received eight unsolicited calls from families wanting to adopt children with AIDS and Peggy's neighbors have invited the girls to play with their children!

The University hospital in Newark, New Jersey has been inundated with AIDS patients. One-third of their general medical beds are now occupied by the AIDS-infected. They are scattered throughout the hospital *and are not identified* (right to privacy).

What state has the most effective laws to combat the AIDS epidemic? Surprisingly, Illinois is way ahead of the other 49. Washington, D.C. is the most backward. The only law on the books in Washington protects homosexuals from discrimination. There are no laws to protect the public in Washington and none are pending. Only Florida, Illinois, and Idaho make it a crime to knowingly infect another person. Other states have legislation in the hopper.

The police in Marietta, Georgia, a suburb of Atlanta, are very upset. By law the hospitals cannot tell police officers whether someone they bring in off the street has AIDS. It would be a violation of the patients' privacy

The Assistant Chief said: "I think everybody—doctors, police, and public are confused." The Chief agrees: "Quite frankly, there's not a lot of information out there and we know so little. Even the medical field doesn't know a lot about the disease."

But the Georgia Board of Education is taking a strong stand.[8] Any teacher or student who shows symptoms of AIDS must submit to an AIDS test. If a teacher refuses he

8 *Wall Street Journal,* 8/25/87.

can be fired, and if a student refuses the test he will be treated as if he had AIDS and taught separately. Georgia is the first state board to adopt such a policy. Shouldn't your state do the same?

Syndicated columnist, Thomas Sowell, said, "The good news is that there is now at least a struggle beginning over whether to protect the public from AIDS-carriers or to protect the AIDS-carriers from the public. The bad news is that the dominant political trend is still to protect those with AIDS instead of the public."[9]

But reality is surfacing in Georgia. Georgia is tied for tenth in the number of reported AIDS cases and a few courageous people are now recommending the obvious. Dr. John D. Watson, Jr., immediate past president of the Medical Association of Georgia, has recommended testing all Georgians over the age of ten and jailing those who refuse to be tested.

"Somewhere down the road," he said, "if a person is supposed to be tested and is not, then he's going to be incarcerated." Now that's the kind of talk we like, using the "I" word—incarcerate those who refuse to cooperate.

Health officials in Georgia said that testing everyone wouldn't be "cost effective." That's baloney. Doctors and hospitals do a test called the SMAC every day in Georgia on thousands of patients. It screens for hepatitis and dozens of other problems. For 50 years hospitals routinely tested all patients admitted to the hospitals for syphilis.

It's not "cost effective" to do a test that might save Western civilization? These health bureaucrats keep harping on "education." Who's left to educate? The American people know what causes AIDS—sexual intercourse with an infected person and many forms of non-sexual contact. We don't need education. We need identification.

---

9 *Marietta Daily Journal,* 8/24/87.

Let's start with checking all prostitutes and drug addicts. Next we should check all hospital personnel and patients and then restaurant employees. To save the next generation, school children should be tested next (and their teachers) and then everybody else including the "health officials" who want to educate this holocaust away.

Susan Hart, infection control officer at Columbus Medical Center, Columbus, Georgia, said that she fears "false positive test results could produce the kind of stigma that may affect a person's employability or ability to get housing." Is Susan willing to risk the demise of our country because of a one in a hundred t0.01) false positive rate with the Western Blot AIDS test?[10]

It is true that the ELISA "screening?' test is worthless, in fact, worse than worthless. A test with a 30 percent or more false positive rate is simply unacceptable. Testing the entire population with this test would lead to chaos. So the ELISA test should be abandoned and the Western Blot test used exclusively until a better test with even fewer false positives is devised. Although the Western Blot is not perfect (no test is), *we must test.*

The homosexual lobby backed up by "liberal" politicians has so much power that they can now have directives passed (things you don't get to vote for or against) that severely punish innocent people for not following Labor Department edicts on AIDS protection. If you are caught not wearing gloves while emptying a bedpan, you can be fined $10,000![11] Anyone in his right mind wouldn't do this kind of work these days without taking precautions. But the person contributing the contents to the bedpan can have AIDS, not tell anyone, and go scot-free.

---

10 Ibid.
11 *New York Times*, 7/23/87.

You think that's crazy? In Fulton County (Atlanta), Georgia, prostitutes testing positive for AIDS are protected from the state criminal justice system. The District Attorney wants to prosecute whores transmitting AIDS but he is not allowed to see test results.[12]

If you just read the headlines you're going to get a lot of disinformation, especially concerning AIDS. A recent article in the *Atlanta Constitution* is typical. The headline read: "AIDS Virus Does Not Make Syphilis Worse, CDC Finds."

But the last paragraph of the article states that the CDC reported on "two patients who progressed to fatal syphilis even though they received penicillin for the disease." Were these patients tested for HTLV-I? HTLV-II? SV-40? What kind of reporting is that? Penicillin-resistant syphilis is unheard of. Why are we seeing it now?

Evidence of the AIDS cover-up continues to surface. CDC statistics would infer that one woman in every one thousand is infected with the AIDS virus. But a study in Alameda County, California, showed an actual infection rate of one in every two hundred women. Alameda County is not San Francisco. It's Yuppie country. The CDC says only 20-30 percent of AIDS-infected persons would get full-blown AIDS. Scientists without a political axe to grind now say that the disease will be 100 percent fatal.

Dr. J. Nicklas Gorden of Georgia Tech University testified before the Georgia State Board of Education. He said that he couldn't understand why the Centers for Disease Control say that AIDS cannot be contracted by "casual contact." As the epidemic reaches "critical mass," casual contact may become the primary method of transmission of the virus.

Frederic Allen really hit the mark in the May 21, 1987, issue of the *Atlanta Constitution:* "No one wishes to see a

---

12 *Atlanta Constitution,* 7/23/87, pg. 1.

white-frocked doctor race out of the CDC's front door screaming 'Plague!,' but the CDC seems to have gone to the opposite extreme. Ever since AIDS burst onto the medical scene ... it has been considered boorish to express fear about the disease. With many in the press joining in, the CDC has established a ministry that delivers a constant sermon: If AIDS scares you, you are intolerant, bigoted, ignorant—a medieval pinhead given to fanciful superstitions."

In California, 20 percent of AIDS deaths are not reported as such. The Liberace-attempted cover-up is typical. His doctor put "heart failure brought on by degenerative brain disease" on the death certificate. I have been in practice for 25 years, and I have never seen anyone die of heart failure from degenerative brain disease. It was a very inept attempt at subterfuge. Liberace died of pneumonia secondary to AIDS. The local coroner insisted on setting the record straight. "I believe," he said, "somebody along the line wanted to pull a fast one on us."

Thirty-nine year old fashion whiz, Willie Smith, has died of "pneumonia," reported the *Atlanta Constitution*. When is the last time you heard of a thirty-nine-year-old dying of pneumonia?

The incredible naiveté of government officials concerning AIDS is awesome. The latest shocker concerns the armed forces. It has been announced that a serviceman may stay in the military even though he tests positive for AIDS if he follows the Army's "guidelines." Not even his wife, much less his buddies, have the right to know that he is infected. The AIDS-infected soldier or sailor is "advised" to inform his wife!

The Pentagon admits that at least 2,500 servicemen are known to be infected. In order to keep our allies from going through the roof about this, the infected servicemen are quietly reassigned to duties in the United States. Pentagon policy is to discharge any service person found to be homosexual, but not those found to have AIDS Unless he is also homosexual. How do they know which ones are and which ones aren't?

Taking confidentiality to the extreme, Colorado recently passed an AIDS law that imposes a $5,000 fine and/or maximum of two years in jail for any physician who informs the patient's spouse or even another doctor to whom the patient is referred that the patient has AIDS.[13]

New York City—The Center of the AIDS Maelstrom

"They Are Fiscally Unprepared For Its Terrible Consequences." That's what the comptroller of New York State said about the public health bureaucrats of New York City. Comptroller, Elinor Bachrach, says that 5,000 AIDS patients will be hospitalized on any given day in New York City by 1991.[14] "These are terrible figures," she said. "We think the public has a right to know and the city has to get prepared for the terrible consequences."

Who's going to pick up New York City's *billion dollars a year* AIDS tab? New York's medicrats want you to: "The real question is whether the government will meet its responsibility . ..."

"When 66-year-old Thelma Richards complained of chest pains and breathing problems last Labor Day, she was rushed to a Bronx emergency department. After several hours of observation and a futile wait for a hospital bed, she was sent home. A few hours later Richards died of a heart attack."[15]

This has become a common occurrence in the New York City area because of the tremendous chaos caused by the AIDS epidemic. It is not at all unusual for patients

---

13 *Int. Med. News,* September 1-14,1987.
14 *New York Times,* 7/23/87.
15 Ibid.

to wait for up to *five days* on a stretcher in the emergency department of a hospital before getting a bed. Government regulations combined with the AIDS problem are nearly *strangling to death* the medical system in our largest city. Even as utilization of beds has skyrocketed, hospital beds have been taken out of service to meet "federal occupancy requirements" and state projections of the number of needed beds.

Twenty-seven percent of the nation's total AIDS patients are located in New York state. It is estimated that AIDS patients will fill 25 percent of all the municipal beds in New York City in the next few years.

Bureaucrats, in all their wisdom, reduced the number of beds in New York City by 2000. "While these beds were removed in a single day," one doctor commented, "the process to restore them when justified by changing utilization patterns can be extremely slow and cumbersome." It can take as long as two years to get them replaced.

"The mechanism for efficient, integrated, organized quality care has broken down throughout the city because our hospitals are full. And that leaves our emergency departments filled to dangerous levels with desperately ill people," comments Dr. Gold Frank of New York.

An anonymous blood sampling of infants born in January of 1988 in New York City reveal that *one out of every 61 babies born in that stare was carrying HIV antibodies.*

Based on this alarming result, New York could see as many as 1,000 infected infants in the year 1988.[16]

Heidi Evans, *New York Times:*

"New York City, 1991. The AIDS plague enters its tenth year.

"The dying wait days for hospital beds. Hundreds of infected babies languish in pediatric wards; the only

---

16 *American Medical New,* 2/12/88.

warm hand they know is the touch of a harried nurse. Prisons and shelters swell with the near dead.

"There is no cure in sight.

"Outside, the AIDS epidemic is cutting the heart out of neighborhoods like Greenwich Village, Harlem and the South Bronx.

"Death toll citywide: 32,000 men, women and children.

"Alive and suffering: 12,600 more.

"Price tag: $1 billion a year in public money.

"That could be the scene three years from now, given how strained the city is in 1988 with half that number of cases."

Governor Robert Martinez, governor of Florida: "AIDS carriers who refuse to stop spreading this fatal disease should no more be allowed to roam free than criminals armed with a deadly weapon."

Mathilde Krim, Ph.D., American Foundation for AIDS Research: "The infection will spread in the general population. The only thing we don't know is at what rate it will happen."

Helen S. Kaplan, M.D.: *The Real Truth About Women and AIDS:* "It is wrong and dangerous to urge women and adolescents to place their futures in condoms to reduce the risks of sexual exposure."[17]

Two hundred dolphins have perished from a disease that appears to be like AIDS. A hitherto innocuous bacterium called vibrio is killing the animals. In the report from the Los Angeles Times (August 20, 1987) there is no mention of a possible AIDS connection, but the evidence is too compelling to be ignored. Like the dolphins, if you get AIDS you can die from a previously innocuous infection such as flu, measles or candida albicans (yeast).

---

17 *AIDS Protection*, September, 1988, Vol. 2, No. 5.

The dolphins died with complications that have an eerie similarity to human AIDS: skin lesions (like Kaposi's sarcoma in humans) and lung parasites (like pneumocystis carini in humans). Dr. Joseph Geraci, a marine pathologist, says, "It seems these animals are presensitized to invasion by bacteria that are otherwise innocuous." That means a weakened immune system. Isn't that AIDS? Why are they ignoring the possible AIDS connection?

Life in the AIDies

- Dr. James Mason of the Centers for Disease Control stated that all blood samples for routine testing at 40 hospitals in 30 states are being routinely tested for AIDS. Representative Henry Waxman of California, asked Mason if he was aware that California has a law that forbids AIDS testing without consent. Mason replied: "Then I sure am committing lots of crimes every day."[18]

- Hollywood is making a multi-million dollar movie claiming AIDS was artificially created by scientists in a laboratory—and says the story is based on fact.[19]

- Dr. Peter Duesberg is so convinced that the AIDS virus doesn't cause AIDS that he is threatening to inject himself with the virus.

- The World Health Organization announced they intend to devote as much effort to eradicating AIDS as they did to eradicating smallpox. In eliminating smallpox they eliminated half the population of Africa with AIDS-contaminated smallpox vaccine. (See Chapter 4.) Maybe we should look elsewhere for help.

---

18 *New York Post*, 3/16/88.
19 *London Sunday Express*, 4/10/88.

- The reported 30,000 cases of AIDS in early 1987 was a pathetically low estimate. The Centers for Disease Control were leaving out many of the worst cases (emaciation and AIDS dementia) because they didn't fit their bureaucratic definition. The CDC has adjusted its statistics which adds almost 8,000 more cases to the Social Security roll. That means $480.00 per month, a housing allowance, and free medical care—$100,000 to $200,000 for each case until dead and buried.

- The American Psychiatric Association has come out strongly *against* mandatory AIDS testing,[20] the only medical specialty to do so.

- In Sacramento, California, three doctors treat 99 percent of the AIDS patients. One of them recently died of AIDS.[21]

- The cancer/AIDS "chemotheraphy" market was over a half billion dollars in 1986 and is expected to hit three quarters of a billion dollars with an average annual growth of over 13 percent. With that kind of profit do you think they will ever find a drug that works?

- A surgeon in Delaware refused to treat a swimmer with a cut foot because of his "homosexual demeanor" and unknown AIDS status.[22]

- In Onandaga County, New York, servers at all restaurant2s3in the county have been ordered to wear plastic gloves.

- A 70-year-old Methodist minister died in the summer of 1987. Bishop Crutchfield had "an unblemished

---

20 *American Medical News*, 7/31/87, p. 3.
21 Op. Cit., p. 28.
22 *Medical Tribune*, 8/5/87.
23 Ibid.

record of service and morality." After his retirement he was active in ministering to people with AIDS—and he died of AIDS. It later turned out that his morality record was far from unblemished.

- A nail salon may refuse an AIDS victim a pedicure because *there is no conclusive evidence on how the dead) disease is spread*, a judge ruled. A West Hollywood, California, ordinance banning AIDS discrimination "fails to respect the right not to be involuntarily exposed to a risk of personal harm," Superior Court Judge Lawrence Waddington said.[24]
- There will be *81,000* patients *blind or going blind* from the complications of AIDS, usually cytomegalovirus infection, by 1991.[25]
- By 1991, according to a *Medical Tribune* report, as many as *10,000* full-time hospital beds will be needed *every day* in New York City for the in-patient care of persons with AIDS.

The President's Message
(The Emergency White House, St. Louis, Missouri, 199?)

"And now, my fellow Americans, I must give you some news that gives me my saddest moment in life, a life that has been bountiful and rewarding. My AIDS is now out of control. I have the strength to continue but, as you know, insanity with paranoia is one of the most common complications of AIDS. The last thing we need with the crisis that is upon us is a paranoid psychotic president.

"To prevent chaos in government I have today signed a directive that orders any cabinet member or other Presidential employee, including all members of the Armed

---

24 *Miami Herald*, 3/26/88.
25 *Medical World News*, 11/23/87.

Forces, to be dismissed immediately when diagnosed as AIDS-positive. We simply cannot afford to have insanity running rife through the arteries of government.

"I have also issued an order that places all transportation, including the airlines, under federal control. This is not a public health measure for, as you know, the virus has spared no region, no city and no racial or religious group. There are simply not enough able-bodied people left to maintain any more than emergency government services. Food and fuel rationing will of course continue for the indefinite future. Because of the worsening problem in the cities, the National Guard has been ordered to shoot looters on sight. AIDS-infected persons having sexual relations, handling food or working in the medical field, except on other AIDS-infected persons, will be placed immediately into the nearest AIDS detention camp for the remainder of their life. The death sentence is to be imposed on all prostitutes, promiscuous persons, intravenous drug users and dealers in drugs.

"Yes, my friends, these measures are unconstitutional in the traditional sense and I deeply regret that the Constitution has been suspended for the duration of this emergency. It is no longer a question of freedom. It is a question of survival of the human race. May God have mercy on us."

The President stared blankly into the camera. Behind his desk the outlines of the Gateway Arch could be seen through the window of the emergency White House. A palpable silence, broken only by the nervous rustling of his papers, fell upon the cramped presidential office. The faint sound of a distant siren suffused through the hot and humid room.

The sound of the siren seemed to bring the President back. He reached into his coat, pulled out a .45 automatic pistol and aimed it directly into the lens of the camera. The explosion smashed the camera into the operator's face, propelling him backward in a mist of blood and glass onto the couch behind him. The President then placed the gun in his mouth and dispatched himself from the presidency.

No one seemed surprised that the President of the United States would do such an outlandish thing. Suicide was an every day reality. AIDS was the number one cause of death followed by suicide. The third highest cause of death was murder-suicide resulting from pacts by dying lovers who were both infected and not interested in witnessing the pain, the puke and the pus of each other's decaying bodies.

Dr. Thrush, with little show of emotion, turned off the television and looked out the window at the empty parking lot. My God, he thought, the President is insane, and maybe dead—what now? He had resisted treating AIDS. He felt he owed it to his patients of 20 years not to risk infecting them by having AIDS patients in the office. But things had changed. You had to treat AIDS. It was not unusual to look out his office window in downtown Atlanta and see someone collapse in the street. The body would lie where it fell until the evening truck came by to cart the dead or dying to a "terminal center" where morphine was given until the breathing stopped. Only two requests were answered in these centers, morphine for pain and water for thirst. The filth had to be largely ignored. There was no one willing or able to care for the toilet needs of thousands of terminal patients.

Those not dying of AIDS were more than likely half-starved because of the chronic food shortages, Dr. Thrush mused, making them even more susceptible to the virus and many other diseases. Dr. Thrush had noted with horror that AIDS was now competing with many other previously controlled infectious diseases. With the breakdown in insect control, public sanitation and the onset of starvation, tuberculosis, yellow fever plague, cholera, syphilis, typhus, malaria and bacterial pneumonia began to vie with the AIDS virus for the title of the Black Knight of the Apocalypse.

Thrush rubbed his eyes, burning from fatigue and cigarette smoke. He pressed the smoldering cigarette butt into the ashtray and rose to leave the deserted office. His staff had left early to attend another funeral.

His wife had objected violently to his resuming smoking. He enjoyed it and was fatalistic. He didn't think that he would live long enough to die of cancer anyway. His wife had died 18 months earlier from a staphylococcus pneumonitis. She did not have AIDS but she was dead just the same. These virulent new bacteria just weren't responding to antibiotics. It was 1790 all over again. Pneumonia, he reminded himself, was an easy way to die.

Thrush rode his motorcycle through the deserted streets of the city, past dimly lit apartments. The smell of kerosene was strong in the humid summer air. The people had not yet been told that the kerosene supplies were dangerously low. When the kerosene was gone, he thought, they would eat raw food and go to bed with the setting sun.

Although he rode a motorcycle out of necessity, he enjoyed it in the summer. The air was instantly cool and it was the only time that he felt free. He was heading home to Myra, in the north Georgia hills.

Myra had moved in when her husband, a policeman, was killed in a food riot. The plague had many lieutenants. You could die of the virus itself or an invading fungus, bacterium, parasite, protozoa, such as malaria, or you could simply die of murder engendered by desperation and the survival instinct. These are part of the legions commanded by The Virus. Murder took Myra's husband. But it was the VIRUS that caused the murder.

As he turned into the driveway of their mountain cabin he saw a dead dog in his path with another emaciated dog eating his flesh. As he approached, the scrawny creature bared his teeth. Without hesitation he drew his .45-caliber automatic and shot the dog in the head.

Dogs had turned wild like land-based sharks. "Better clean *that* mess up in a hurry," he thought, "or we'll have a feeding frenzy on our hands."

He parked his bike and headed for the house. Myra hadn't been well lately. He wondered....

Chapter 4
The Origin of AIDS

The world was startled when the *London Times* reported on its front page, May 11, 1987, that the World Health Organization (WHO) had "triggered" the AIDS epidemic in Africa through the WHO smallpox immunization program. The only people in the free world not surprised by the *London Times* front page expose were the Americans—because they never heard about it. It is chilling to think that our press is so controlled that the most momentous news break since the assassination of President Kennedy didn't even make the sports section, much less the front page of *any American daily paper; radio or television news.*

A careful study of World Health Organization (VVHO) literature reveals the careful planning that went into the seeding of AIDS in various nations.[1]

"A systematic evaluation of the effects of viruses on immune functions should be undertaken.... An attempt should be made to ascertain whether viruses can in fact exert selective effects on immune function. . . by affecting T-cell function as opposed to B-cell function. The possibility should also be looked into *that the immune response to the virus itself may be impaired* if the infecting virus damages more or less selectively the cells responding to the viral antigen...."

You don't have to know much virology to see that as a clear call to scientists to attempt to make an immune-destroying virus, an acquired immune deficiency—AIDS.

---

1   *Bul.* WHO, Vol. 47,1972, pp.257-274.

They also laid out a modus operandi for their diabolical scheme:[2]

"In the relation to the immune response a *number of useful experimental approaches can be visualized.* " They suggested that a neat way to do this would be to put their new killer virus (AIDS) into a vaccination program, sit back and observe the results. "This would be particularly informative in sibships," they said. That is, give the AIDS virus to brothers and sisters and see if they die, who dies first, and of what, just like using rats in a laboratory.

They used smallpox vaccine for their vehicle and the geographical sites chosen in 1972 were Uganda and other African states, Haiti and Brazil. *The recent past of AIDS epidemiology coincided with these geographical areas.*

To understand the enormity of our betrayal you must know about the origin of the AIDS virus. The virologists of the world, the sorcerers who brought us this ghastly plague, have formed a united front in denying that the virus was laboratory-made from known, lethal animal viruses. The scientific party line is that a monkey in Africa with AIDS bit a native on the butt. The native then went to town and gave it to a prostitute who gave it to the local banker who gave it to his wife and three girl friends and wham—75 million people became infected with AIDS in Africa. An entirely preposterous story.

Dr. Robert Gallo, "the co-discoverer of the AIDS virus," was interviewed by *Newsweek* for their "On Health" special issue (Fall, 1987).

In the *Newsweek* article Gallo continued to obfuscate by reiterating the disproven green monkey theory. Gallo knows perfectly well that AIDS was spread in Africa and around the world by the AIDS-contaminated smallpox vaccine of the World Health Organization. Being a mem-

2 *Federation Proc. of the U.S.,* Vol. 31, #3, May-June, 1972.

ber of their team and, at least indirectly, paid by them and the National Institute of Health (NIH), he is trying to pin the blame on the green monkey and *16th-century Portuguese traders*.

Gallo continues to spread confusion and disinformation among scientists and the public. Through his influence, and the influence of others in the U.S. bureaucratic Establishment, AIDS research was thrown back at least a year. Gallo knows that AIDS and HTLV-I didn't exist in nature before about 1970. Gallo knows that these viruses are laboratory viruses.

Monkeys don't get it and humans, including Portuguese traders, don't get it until it has been manufactured in a lab and run through human tissue cells. Or in the case of monkeys, run though monkey tissue cells. If there were any virologists in Portugal engineering these viruses during the 16th century it is the best-kept secret in the annals of medical history.

Next Gallo appeared on *60 Minutes* (the guy's everywhere). "All the scientific signposts point to Africa," the *60 Minutes* commentator said in introducing Gallo on November 8, 1987.

"No one can prove where AIDS began," Dr. Gallo says, "[but] if monkeys in central Africa harbor retroviruses, and they do; and if some of them are like the human leukemia virus, and they are; and if some of them are like the human AIDS virus, and they are; and if monkeys when they are caught sometimes bite, and I think they do, then doesn't it make reasonable sense that is the best bet until someone comes up with a better idea?"

The answer is that anyone could come up with a better idea because:

• Many animals "harbor retroviruses," including rats, sheep, cattle and pigs, but none of them has ever appeared in man until recently.

80

- These viruses are all like the human leukemia virus except AIDS which is cytocidal and not leukemic, i.e., it kills the T-cells rather than causing a multiplication of these cells as in leukemia.

- Few of them are "like an AIDS virus" except for being in the retrovirus family.

- The fact that monkeys sometimes bite is irrelevant. Cats and pigs bite too, but they don't transmit AIDS. Only humans transmit AIDS to humans because cats, pigs and monkeys don't get AIDS. The human virus is not pathogenic in animals[3] and the various monkey viruses are not associated with disease in wild animals[4] except when laboratory-induced after capture.

- There has never been a proven case of a monkey transmitting a retrovirus to a human by bite or otherwise. Even monkeys artificially given AIDS by injection do not transmit the disease even to other monkeys.

- AIDS started in the cities of Africa where there are no wild monkeys, not in the villages.

- The doubling time of AIDS infection, being about 12 months, means that one monkey biting one native and then spreading the disease throughout Africa would have taken 20 years to reach a million cases. Seventy-five millions Africans became infected *practically simultaneously. At the same time* the disease became rampant in the U.S., Haiti and Brazil. How could one monkey do that, even if he were an international flight attendant?

---

3 Duesberg, "Cancer Res." 47, 1199-1220, 3/1/87.
4 Ibid.
5 Quinn, T. C., Mann, J.M., "AIDS in Africa: an Epidemiologic Paradigm," Science, 234-955,1986.

81

As Dr. Robert Strecker said on a KPFK Los Angeles radio show, "If you want to listen to the so-called experts for the truth in this disease we'll all be dead."

How many cats have feline acquired immune deficiency syndrome (FAIDS)? Many. How many cats have bitten humans? Many. How many humans have caught AIDS from cats? None.

Duesberg states categorically that, "The human (AIDS) virus is not pathogenic to animals" and the monkey viruses "are never associated with a disease in wild animals."[6] Furthermore, animal AIDS, such as FAIDS and sheep visna, are not transmitted to humans.

I'm finally getting some help from the virology experts in exonerating the green monkey. "The popular theory that the AIDS virus jumped the biologic gap from the African green monkey to man drew nothing but scorn at an international conference on AIDS in Africa," reports *Internal Medicine News*, volume 20, No. 24.

Ironically, the conference was presented by the World Health Organization, the people who contaminated Africa with AIDS through smallpox vaccine. (No one mentioned that at the conference.)

Dr. Luc Montagnier, the real discoverer of the AIDS virus said, "There is no evidence of any reservoir species of monkeys that is truly positive for HIV (AIDS)."

A lot of misconceptions about AIDS were cleared up at this meeting but I doubt you'll hear about it on the evening news. The injecting of monkey blood for ritual purposes is probably a myth, long-time African experts reported. And contrary to popular belief, *AIDS is not found in the rural areas where they hunt, eat and get bitten by monkeys but, almost exclusively in the cities where they have no exposure to monkeys.*

---

6 Ibid.

Dr. Peter Piot, an African AIDS expert from Belgium, said, "The biologic gap between the monkey virus and human host is too wide to be bridged *in a single step* even with direct injection of blood."

I emphasized "in a single step" in the quotation above because it takes *many* steps in a laboratory to engineer an animal virus to infect humans. AIDS is an animal virus, probably bovine visna virus, adapted for man. *It was no accident.*

Where does that leave Gallo's monkey business? His monkey would have to be taken from Africa, inoculated at the Fort Detrick, Maryland, laboratory (or similar sorcerer's workshop), and then taken back to Africa to bite a few million people—if monkeys transmitted AIDS to humans in the first place, which they don't.

Gallo next pops up in *American Medical News*, 12/4/87. He got a five-page spread with no less than six pictures of himself, mostly in color. The headline for the article is simple, half-inch bold type: **"ROBERT C. GALLO, M.D."** Talk about adulation.

The reporter at least had the courage to ask Gallo about his claim to have discovered the AIDS virus when in fact the French at the Pasteur Institute had isolated it a year earlier. Somehow the photos of the virus taken by the French ended up in Gallo's article announcing his momentous discovery.

When found out, Gallo said it was simply a mistake of some sort, the whole thing was just "baked-over media hype" and he was perfectly willing to give the French half the credit. Some gall.

The one thing Gallo said in this interview that I'm sure I agree with was: "Who the hell knows exactly how this virus spread?" (I'm going to tell the green monkey he said that.)

Genetically A1DS (HIV-I) is not even close to the monkey form of immuno-deficiency virus.[7] The genetic structure of any living organism is arranged in what is called codons: triplicates of amino acid "base pairs." These base pairs, composed of the amino acids adenine, guanine, thiamine, cytosine, etc. are the basic structure and identification system of all life, similar you might say, to a print board of a computer.

If you study these various amino acid combinations in the codon, you can identify absolutely what that particular organism is. You can definitely say that it is a rat or a rabbit or it's from a cabbage or an oak tree. No two codons in any living thing are the same. Example I below has a codon obviously different from example II. Consequently, we know that they are from different living species.

Example # I:

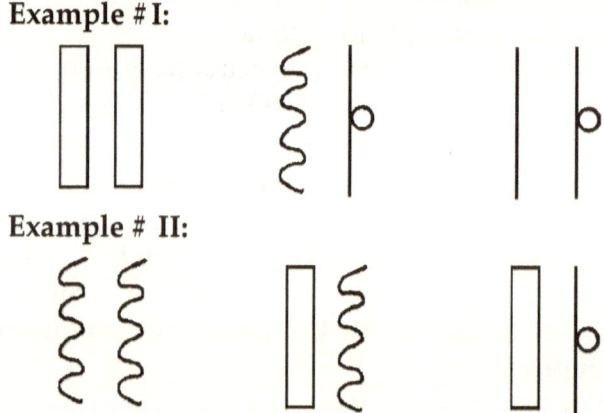

Example # II:

The codons of AIDS do not exist in monkeys or other primates. The message encoded in the base pairs of AIDS does not come from monkeys—it's impossible: not improbable—*impossible.*

---

7 Ibid.

Much of the codon from AIDS would exist in primates (monkeys, apes, etc.), if it came from primates. The AIDS codon exists only in bovine (cattle) leukemia virus, sheep visna virus, cauliflower mosaic virus, and a few others. The "language" or the "print-out" of the DNA, i.e. the base pairs, is entirely different from the language of the DNA in monkeys, apes, man, etc.

Consequently, we know beyond a shadow of a doubt that the AIDS virus came from a combination of cattle and sheep and simply had to be a genetically engineered virus in a laboratory. Gallo knows this. Essex and Haseltine know this. How long will they be able to keep the lid on this cover-up of the crime of the millennium?

Japanese researchers punched more holes in the monkey bite theory of the origin of AIDS and confirmed that it doesn't make any scientific sense. They have studied the entire genetic code of the AIDS-like virus that infects African green monkeys and have concluded that it would be impossible for green monkeys to be the source of AIDS.[8]

It is obvious that one monkey couldn't have caused AIDS (or one homosexual either). *There had to be some sort of simultaneous seeding process.* The only worldwide simultaneous seeding going on at the time was the smallpox vaccine program of the World Health Organization, the WHO. The early epidemiology of the AIDS pandemic fits the smallpox vaccination project of the WHO and nothing else (with the exception of the U.S. which we will explain subsequently).

The AIDS virus was created in a laboratory by combining lethal animal "retroviruses" in human cancer (HeLa) cell cultures and/or calf serum. (See Chapter 6.) These *viruses have never before caused infections in man.* The "species barrier" has always been nature's way of keeping

8 Orange County Register, Wednesday, 6/8/88

85

a deadly virus from wiping out the entire animal kingdom, including man. The myxoma virus of rabbits, for example, wiped out the rabbit population of Europe, but man and other animals were not affected. The sheep visna virus completely decimated the Hocks of Iceland, but no other animal was affected.

The virologists deny that the AIDS virus, HIV-I, is of animal origin. I am sure that you see the paradox here. Aren't monkeys animals?

They are also united in saying that it's not possible for the virus to have been engineered in a laboratory. If it didn't come from other animals and it didn't come from a laboratory and they now admit privately that the monkey couldn't have done it, then it must have come out of thin air. That's a theological position and hence beyond argument. It's certainly not scientific.

These scientists, creating deadly viruses in their sorcerer's retrovirology laboratories, are constantly caught in their own lies. The line goes: "The AIDS virus could not have been engineered in a laboratory because the technology wasn't available until recently." Icelandic scientists combined the sheep visna virus with human tissue cells *over 20years ago*. The technology has been refined in recent years, but the basic process has been actively used in labs all over the world for long before the AIDS virus made its dramatic appearance.

But the scientists hold fast in their denial of culpability.

Professor William Jarrett said, when asked about the possibility of AIDS arising from animal retroviruses, "That is like someone saying babies come out of cabbages."[9]

Dr. Robert Gallo said that people who claim AIDS was manufactured artificially are "either insane or communists."[10]

9 Private communication, John Seale, M.D., 1988.
10 Ibid.

Dr. J. Weiss: "Anyone who says AIDS came from a laboratory is either anti-science or a vivisectionist."

Dr. Luis Montagnier, the discoverer of the AIDS virus, said, "In 1970 there was not enough knowledge in genetic engineering to make such a virus starting from already existing viruses."[11] (See Icelandic experiments mentioned above).

This tower of lies must eventually fall of its own weight. Then what? Where do we look for a solution? Certainly not from the people who caused the disaster. But where—the Pentagon? *The Pentagon is supporting research on biological warfare in over 100 Federal and private laboratories including many prominent universities.*[12] Yet, Neil Levitt, who worked for 17 years at the Army's Infectious Disease Institute, says, "It's a joke... there's no defense against these kinds of organisms. And if you can't defend against something, then why are we pouring more and more money into it? There's something else going on that we don't know about."[13]

Some joke.

Alert readers will say, we don't give smallpox vaccinations in the U.S., so how do you explain the simultaneous outbreak of AIDS in Africa, Brazil and Haiti, where they did indeed give the vaccine, with the U.S. where they didn't give the vaccine?

Simple. *The homosexual community was used as a large group of experimental animals* through the hepatitis-B program. It didn't take many infected homosexuals among the I.V. drug users to quickly spread the disease among a large percentage of the addicts due to the near certainty of infection through direct intravenous insertion of the virus.

---

11 First International Conference on the Global Impact of AIDS, London, March 8-10,1988.
12 *New Scientist, London,* 5/19188.
13 *Science News,* 133:100, 2/13188.

To understand the seeding of AIDS among homosexuals, (and eventually to the rest of us through bisexuals unless drastic action is taken), you must know about a character with the strange name of Wolf Szmuness. His life story will seem bizarre to you unless, like me, you have a conspiratorial turn of mind.

Dr. Szmuness was a Polish jew who supposedly ended up in a Siberian labor camp during World War II. But after the war he somehow became a privileged person, was sent to medical school in Tomsk, Russia, and married a Russian woman, hardly typical treatment of an enemy of the Soviet state.

Szmuness' biographer said that Wolf was always reluctant to discuss "those dark years in Siberia." Maybe he was reluctant because he wasn't in Siberia. If he was he certainly wasn't shoveling salt.

In 1959 the Soviet government "allowed" him to practice in Poland in a public health capacity.

Standard policy in all Communist countries is never to allow all members of a family to travel out of the country to the West at the same time. This eliminates 98 percent of all defection attempts. I have physician friends in Hungary, for example. *He* can go to a meeting anywhere in the world if she stays home. She can go if he stays home. They can both go if the *children* are left at home.

But in 1969, the entire Szmuness family was allowed by communist Poland to go to a medical meeting in Italy. At that time they "defected" and moved to New York City.

With no American credentials whatsoever, he immediately got a job as a "lab technician" at the New York: City Blood Center. Within a very few years this Polish immigrant was given his own lab, a separate department of epidemiology was created for him at the blood bank and he, like the chrysalis turning into a butterfly, changed into *a full professor of epidemiology at the Columbia Medical School!*

In six years this "lab tech" became a full professor *and then went back to Moscow* for a scientific presentation and was received as a dignitary, not a defector.

We tell you this amazing story because in retrospect it is obvious that Wolf Szmuness was a carefully groomed communist agent, planted here after years of preparation, to instigate biological warfare against the American people.

Szmuness, *with the full cooperation and financial support of the US. Centers for Disease Control and the National Institutes of Health,* masterminded the hepatitis-B vaccine experimental program used on homosexual men. He insisted that only young, promiscuous homosexuals be allowed to participate in the experiment. The experiment started in New York at the blood bank in November, 1978. The experimental vaccine was produced in a government-supervised laboratory.[14]

The study was completed in October, 1979. *Within 10 years most of these young men would be dead or dying from AIDS.*

In 1980 the program was expanded to major cities all across the U.S. In the fall of 1980 the first AIDS case was reported in San Francisco. Eight years later most of the homosexuals in San Francisco were infected, dead or dying.

Szmuness did not live to see the fruition of this larger experiment. He died of cancer in 1982.

In 1986 Dr. Cladd Stevens, one of Szmuness' collaborators, penned an astonishing report that did not make your local newspaper. She reported that the majority of the homosexuals in the experimental program were infected with the AIDS virus.[15] The AIDS-laced vaccine, through the bridge of bi-sexual men, now infects as many as three million Americans.

Mission accomplished.

---

14 Cantwell, AIDS and the Doctors of Death, Aries
    Rising Press, Los Angeles, pp.76.
15 Op. Cit., Joklik, pp. 36.

89

Chapter 5
Brave New World—Brave New Bugs

Many people expressed concern when scientists first split the atom. But the splitting of the atom brought us many wonderful things: atomic energy, new medical diagnostic techniques, heretofore unthinkable space projects, and the atomic bomb. Now scientists are splitting something far closer to home than the average atom—the human gene pool.

By using a certain type of enzyme called "restriction enzymes" scientists can now take the DNA compound, which actually composes life itself, and create new bugs, new life forms—and possibly new monsters.

With this momentous step in science, we are embarking on a vast dark ocean far more threatening than what Columbus faced in the fifteenth century. Mankind is floating in a little boat under the control of egotistical, naive, ambitious, greedy, materialistic and irresponsible geneticists and microbiologists who care not for the fate of the human race, but only for their own glory.

As Dr. Irwin Chargaff has said, "What can be done, must be done."

These arrogant scientists have created cancer-causing viruses. They have done many strange things such as combining human cells with genes of the tobacco plant-a combination of vegetable and animal to create something that God did not intend.

Scientists have taken the naive attitude that all knowledge must have a positive result and a good end point. Can this be said of an experiment in Japan where they are mating a woman with a monkey? Is it a good "end point" to mix cobra venom genes with the bacterium E. coli, which is found in the gut of every human being on earth, in order to produce a cobra venom-producing bacterium within your own body? The prospect of all this is certainly intriguing, exciting, irresistible—and terrifying. Frankenstein Lives!

June Goodfield was remarkably prescient when she said in 1977:

"Had the recent work in molecular biology been as innocent a problem as the number of lichens accommodated on a church spire, or abstract as the number of angels upon the head of a pin, the social questions about the impact of science could rumble on like distant thunder, ignored by most scientists who, happily minding their own business, have rarely troubled to lift their heads from the bench. But these bugs are neither innocent nor abstract. The potential dangers maybe enormous, *they may be highly pathogenic, cause epidemics or even pandemics, in humans. They may spread into many new environments and cause great ecological damage. They may cause cancer. No one really knows.*"[1] (Emphasis added.)

Yet Dr. David Baltimore, a scientist who should know better, has said, "Scientists must educate the public not to fear experiments with genetically altered animals or plants or organisms."

Like most scientists with egos larger than life (especially those who have won Nobel prizes like Baltimore), he follows this arrogant statement with the usual political rhetoric. He declares that there should be "an end to star wars" and, of course, no cooperation with the government in research on biological weapons to counter the Soviets who have openly admitted that they are stockpiling such weapons and creating ever new and more powerful ones.

The warnings have been clear and consistently given by many responsible scientists. Dr. Michael Thomas, a

---

1 Goodfield, **Playing God**, Random House, Inc., New York, 1977.

member of the British Medical Association's Board of Science, warned that genetic engineering could produce cancer *and even endanger the survival of the human race.* He said, "The danger is that by trying to treat and eradicate disease by... gene therapy, we may so deplete the genetic gene pool that there will be no chance variations available to survive future environmental challenges."[2]

Perhaps the best illustration of the biological terror that is being let loose upon us is the recent finding at the Center for Health Science, University of California at Los Angeles.[3] Scientists at UCLA inoculated mice simultaneously with two strains of herpes simplex virus type 1 (the common cold sore). Each of these viruses has a very weak ability to invade nerve tissue and so singly they are considered harmless. But they found that when the two weak viruses were combined, they had created a new and very deadly viral recombinant.

The reason, the scientists reported, for the extreme virulence of the newly created life form is that the two viruses exchange genetic material to produce the killer offspring. The new virus was so deadly that even when painted on the foot of a mouse he quickly died! Dosages of the original, harmless viruses, 100 times more concentrated than the recombinant virus, had no deleterious effect on the animals.

There is a very important message here. When virologists shotgun viruses into tissue cultures and create new germs, or when they mate two viruses as in this herpes case, they have no idea what kind or how many Frankenstein monsters they are creating. As many scientists have warned, because of these incredible experiments, the human race may be on the verge of extinction.

---

2 AP, 2/20/88.
3 R. Javier, Biotechnology News, 12/10/86.

J. Clemmensen said in 1975,[4] "We have in tissue cultures created conditions for propagating virus in cells from a host different from the original. This will tend to increase enormously the chance of mutation into variants acceptable to new hosts, and by their heterogenic qualities they may have neoplastic (cancerous) capacity in a new host. *So it is possible to visualize a mutation of a virus into a variety of high contagiosity to man resulting in a pandemic of neoplastic disease before we can develop a vaccine.*" (Emphasis added.)

Public hearings in Cambridge, Massachusetts, concerning the new life-creating science of recombinant genetic engineering brought out some startling facts concerning the laboratories at Harvard University. It was revealed that the laboratories are infested with red ants and cockroaches which have resisted all efforts of modern science to eliminate them. These creatures can carry radioactivity from the laboratories and the various terrible germs that scientists are manipulating and creating there. If the geniuses at Harvard cannot contain cockroaches and ants, it has been asked, then how can they be expected to contain invisible, deadly microbes in their "high security" laboratories?

To understand the mentality and mindset of many of today's microbiologists and geneticists it is necessary to look at the man who formed the minds of so many of today's biological scientists: Dr. Charles B. Davenport.

As America's leading eugenicist, Davenport's ideas emanating from his fiefdom at Cold Spring Harbor, New York, had a cataclysmic effect on the thinking of the men who are dealing with these various experiments today. Davenport, working with tens of millions of dollars from the Carnegie Institute, was without question the godfa-

---

4   Danish Cancer Register, 1975.

ther of all of these biological madmen working in laboratories today around the world.

Charles Davenport, the father of human eugenics, felt that the American race needed improvement through what he called "negative eugenics," the preventing of reproduction by the genetically defective, possibly by state enforced sterilization. If the state could take a person's life, Davenport reasoned, surely it could deny the lesser right of reproduction. Davenport said "The most progressive revolution in history could be achieved by placing human matings on the same high plane as that of horse breeding."

Of course not all contemporary scientists went along with Davenport's desire to play God. Dr. Pearson said "The success of these things always lies in the individual who dominates the whole, and our friend Davenport is not a clear strong thinker."

Dr. Davenport was devoutly anti-Semitic. Jews show "the greatest proportion of offenses against chastity in connection with prostitution, the lowest of crimes." He was violently and emotionally anti-sex and even advocated drastic measures to suppress it. He was a strong supporter of sterilization of those of whom he did not approve but stated that castration should be used instead of vasectomy in males because it "cuts off the hormones and makes the patient docile, tractable and without sex desire."

Davenport, perhaps more prescient than he realized, once stated, "It is going to be a purifying *conflagration* someday!" (Emphasis in the original.) Davenport was a piece of work alright. Hitler would have loved him.

The Global 2000 Committee, which wants to eradicate billions of people, for the common good of course, is merely an extension of the ideas of Davenport. The enormous influence of Dr. Davenport on the work at Cold Spring Harbor and the thinking of geneticists-and even

94

high school students—is beyond exaggeration. Cold Spring Harbor, New York, may be the epicenter for the genetic bomb that will eradicate mankind. Much of the original genetic engineering that led to the present AIDS holocaust was done at Cold Spring Harbor, referred to by those in the know as "Camp Cancer."

You probably have an image of highly trained scientists wearing space suits and working in closely guarded laboratories as the only people engaged in this risky business of creating new (and often dangerous) life forms. This image is incorrect.

Fifteen-year-old kids are now creating new bacteria in ordinary high school laboratories at Cold Spring Harbor high school.[5] It's called "bacterial transformation." It's deceptively simple with the high tech equipment now available to students. They are using E. coli, the germ that is a normal inhabitant in the gut of every human being, the one scientists have been warning *other scientists* to be careful of because of the potential for contamination of the human gene pool.

"These are very content cells," says Mark Bloom, education director at the school. "We're going to change that soon."

They may change a lot of things.

Elko, South Carolina, population 202, is not a community one would expect to have national, international and historic significance. There's no Chamber of Commerce, no symphony and no 5 P.M. traffic reports. It's what reporters would call "a sleepy little southern town." But Elko may become as well known as Chernobyl, Alamagordo (New Mexico), and Hiroshima. Alamagordo only produced an atomic bomb. Elko may produce a biological bomb.

---

5 N.Y. Times. 3/24/88

On a misty fall morning in 1987, three miles from Elko, scientists in heavy protective gear including goggles and rubber gloves, worked quietly behind a heavily guarded compound. An 8-foot electrified fence, flood lights and armed guards—sounds like a concentration camp, but it's only scientists from Clemson University sowing man-made recombinant (genetically altered) bacteria into a field of winter wheat.

This will be the first "outdoor" test of genetically-altered bacteria containing genes from another bacterium. I put the word "outdoor" in quotes because the genetically altered smallpox vaccine, used to decimate 75,000,000 Africans with AIDS, went directly into people rather than being sprayed on crops. (Maybe they didn't think of spraying crops.)

Some scientists are very concerned about this. This man-manipulated bacterium turns blue when it eats lactose sugar. Lactose is the sugar in dairy products. Will you turn blue when this new bacteria in your bread enters your body and combines with milk or other lactose-containing foods?

Joe Wilder isn't concerned. Mr. Wilder is a legislator from Barnwell. He said: "It would be a mistake to think that we are ignorant people who don't know what is going on. Certain types of genetic engineering could be disastrous or could be detrimental. But we are talking about a microbe here that is innocuous."[6] (Keep in mind that a single bacterium will make *a few billion* copies of itself *ovenight*.)

The Environmental Protection Agency, Clemson University, most virologists, the mouthpiece of government medicine known as the National Academy of Sciences, *The Wall Street Journal* and Williston, South Carolina, high school teacher Joe Moseley all agree with M. Wilder. Mr.

6   Atlanta Constitution, 10/31/87.

Moseley said, (emphasis added) "*If* all we have been told is true, the test will be *pretty well* contained." (Is "pretty well" good enough?)

Let's leave bucolic Elko, South Carolina, and look in on the world of the geneticists and retro-virologists. We'll return later to Elko.

Around 1972 scientists developed a method for *mixing genes at will from any two or more organisms on earth.* The genes of a duck can be mixed with the genes of an orange or a zebra. Thus far we haven't seen any quacking fruit or duck-billed zebras but it's not due to lack of effort by scientists playing God.

When viruses and bacteria are used in these gene transfers they may enter your body to become part of your *permanent genetic makeup.* Theoretically these genes, whether they are from snake, rabbit, a deadly virus such as AIDS, cauliflower or broccoli, can be transmitted to your progeny. Most of us would not want broccoli in our family tree; snake or rabbit either.

Dr. Robert Pollack, a respected cancer researcher, is nervous about all this. In fact, he's *been* nervous for 15years. Back in the 70's Pollack took issue with scientists who were making SV-40 virus in large batches. Virologists like SV-40 because it's a very simple organism and thus easily manipulated. But it causes cancer in humans.

Pollack's anxiety dramatically increased when at a meeting in Cold Spring Harbor biochemist Janet Mertz proudly announced that she and her colleagues at Stanford intended to combine genetically the SV-40 virus with the bacterium E coli.

Your anxiety level is about to go up too. E. coli is the major organism in your intestinal tract. Trillions of these bacteria live in peace in the colon of every human being. What, Pollack asked, will happen if E. coli genetically combined with SV-40 is turned loose in the general population—and into your gut?

If the experiment were to be carried out how could contamination be prevented? Polio vaccine, hepatitis-B vaccine and smallpox vaccine have caused hundreds of cases of severe illness, paralysis and even death. Although it has never been admitted, many of these tragedies were probably caused by a polio-like virus contaminant. The record is not good.

For once, scientists listened to the doomsayers and plans at Stanford University for combining E. coli and SV 40 were dropped. They went further. A group of leading scientists submitted a letter to Science and Nature magazine which was published in July, 1974. The letter called for scientists to:

- *not* improve the resistance of germs to antibiotics,
- *not* to combine animal viruses such as SV-40 with bacteria and
- *not* to combine genes for deadly toxins into organisms.

Scientists were asked to defer indefinitely all experiments involving genes from bacteria or viruses dangerous to people. Dr. Berg of Stanford was pleased with their report. "I think we have planted the seed," he said. But the fruit proved very bitter.

It wasn't long before "shotgun experimentation" was invented, a form of genetic Russian roulette. Shotgun genetic experiments are done by taking an organism, say a malaria parasite, and chopping up the DNA into many small segments containing a few genes each. These segments are then separately inserted into a germ such as E. coli and mass-produced. A scientist couldn't be accused of dealing with known deadly genes. He simply wouldn't know what he was dealing with until after it was accomplished.

These scientific sorcerers have created new forms of life. Which of the Great Powers will direct them? Even former advocates of recombinant engineering are having second thoughts. Dr. Robert Sinsheimer of Cal Tech said, "I thought of very careful experiments to replace gene A with gene B. It never occurred to me that someone would do a shotgun experiment."

Nobel prize winner George Wald has sounded a warning from Harvard: "Our ignorance is profound," he said and he pointed out that new and old diseases are constantly appearing *without* man's interference. With man's interference they are certain to multiply. "If the worst happened under this recombinant DNA research you'd never be able to identify the disease, still less trace it to its source. It would be just a mystery."

Dr. Shaw Livermore of the University of Michigan attempted to block laboratory genesis at his university: "It should not demean man to say that we may now be unable to manage successfully a capability for altering life itself." His was a lonely voice falling on the wet ears of young Turks eager to get on with their new toys and create their share of new life in the laboratory.

Dr. F. M. Burnett, a pioneer in the field of microbiology, wrote a grim warning to the world over 20years ago:[7] "It seems almost indecent to hint that, so far as the advancement of medicine is concerned, molecular biology may be an evil thing The human implications of what is going on... are at best dubious, at worst terrifying"

Burnett points out that genetic manipulation of viruses appears to have only negative results, i.e., anti-life functions. "For the foreseeable future," he said, "the only function of viruses is to destroy higher forms of life." And, he points out, experiments in viral genetics "... could grow into the almost unimaginable catastrophe of a 'virgin-soil' epidemic... involving all the populous regions of the world."

---

7 Lancet, 1/1/66.

With our hindsight we can now see this as a clear prediction, given over 20 years ago, of the present AIDS pandemic.

Again with our hindsight we can see where Dr. Burnett underestimated man's capacity for evil. In discussing the use of malignant cells in tissue cultures he said, "It is highly unlikely that the use of malignant cells . . . as a subtle means of homicide could ever be developed." But, revealing a certain ambivalence, he added, "Practical applications of molecular biology to cancer research might also be sinister—they are not likely to be helpful. It is hard for an experimental scientist to accept," he concluded, "but it is becoming all too evident that there are dangers in knowing what should not be known. But no one has ever heeded the words of a Cassandra."

And now back to Elko, South Carolina. It turns out that the bacterium chosen for this gene splicing experiment which is being sprayed on a remote South Carolina wheat field *is none other than E. coli, the bug that lives in your gat, the one Pollack was concerned might escape from a laboratory after being combined with cancer genes.*

We are assured by all of those august organizations mentioned earlier that this experiment being conducted behind electrified barbed wire is perfectly safe and of course there is no risk of cancer-causing germs developing as a result.

These reassurances are not reassuring in the light of the facts concerning the genetic engineering technology involved. *Purified genes depend on materials derived from cancer viruses* and cancer cells. The medium for cell culture is usually calf serum. *Calf serum is very common) contaminated with bovine leukemia virus* which causes T-cell leukemia in man.[8] The UCLA report concerning combin-

---

8 In Viro, Vol. 11, #6,1975.

ing innocuous organisms (see pp. 94) clearly warns of the danger in the Elko and similar experiments.

Mad Scientists and the HeLa Monster

Henrietta Lacks is a black woman you need to know about. Like Jesus Christ she died in her early 30's and became the first person since Jesus to become immortal, in a cellular sense.

Scientists have been trying to grow human tissue cells in the laboratory with no success for most of the 20th century. In February, 1951, an unnoticed cataclysmic event took place which changed science forever—Henrietta Lacks entered Johns Hopkins University Hospital in Baltimore, Maryland.

Henrietta, a Baltimore housewife, had cancer of the cervix, not just any cancer but a vicious fire storm of a cancer that consumed her in a few months. But a part of Henrietta did not die. Soon after her diagnosis was made a surgeon snipped off a piece of the cancerous tissue from her cervix, put it in some calf serum culture medium and watched with utter amazement as it began to grow like psycho crab grass—breakthrough, immortal human tissue cells! They grew so fast that they were able to *double their number every 24 hours—a million cells today, a quadrillion by a week from next Tuesday.*

This was a dream-come-true for the microbiologists. So what that they were incredibly malignant; cells are cells and science must march on. There are studies to be done, grants to be gotten, viruses to be manufactured and Nobel prizes to be won.

Let's jump forward 20 years. (Henrietta will be back.) In 1972, an election year, President Richard Nixon declared his "War on Cancer" and "persuaded" the Russians (Why the Russians? Why not the French or Germans?) to join in this great crusade. To show our sincerity (we're always showing the Russians our "sincerity") we sent a delegation of crazy American cancer researchers to Moscow and presented *their crazy* cancer researchers with a cute gold-lettered box containing 30 cancer-causing animal viruses. (At least they *thought* they were only animal viruses.)

What harm could such an impressive gesture of good will do? After all they were only animal cancer viruses which had never been proven to cause cancer in humans. The Russians, always wanting to one-up the Americans, presented their guests with six human cell cultures from six different cancer victims from six different parts of Russia. The cultures, the Russians said, contained *human* cancer causing viruses.

Remarkable. The American scientists had not found one genuine human cancer virus much less six. Were the Russians pulling our leg again? No one dared challenge this incredible breakthrough. It wouldn't be polite. It would damage East-West relations.

Our government turned the six Russian viral cell cultures over to Dr. Walter A. Nelson-Rees, a highly respected San Francisco geneticist, for safe-keeping. He was not instructed to examine them, which seems rather strange, only to store them. But a top scientist like Nelson-Rees isn't about to just stare at his refrigerator when it is said to contain the world's first identi5~ed human cancer virus-containing cells.

He popped them under the microscope and immediately noticed a peculiar thing. There were no Y chromosomes, only X, meaning that all six cases were from females. Well, that could happen.

He sent the six specimens to Ward Peterson, a Detroit enzymologist and asked him to study them enzymatically. Each specimen contained an enzyme called G6PD *which is found only in the negro race.* Six cultures from *six black females* in Russia? Are there six black females in Russia? There is no indigenous negro population in the Soviet Union and blacks are not allowed to immigrate to the socialist paradise. Remember G6PD. It will, like Henrietta, return again.

The puzzle was taking shape. Next Nelson-Rees called a colleague in Washington and asked him to check out the "human cancer virus" ostensibly in these cells. Dr. Wade Parks reported that the only virus present in the cells of the six specimens was a monkey virus which wasn't a cancer virus but a worthless contaminant.

With this report Nelson-Rees popped the question to Parks: "Has it occurred to you that these cells may all be from the same patient?" Yes, Parks said, it had occurred to him.

Nelson-Rees had his suspect cornered. All that remained to clinch the case was in his department— detailed chromosome examination through a staining process called purple banding.

The conclusion was inescapable. Henrietta Lacks was living and well in Washington, Detroit, Moscow, San Francisco and points in between. Henrietta, who probably never left Baltimore, was a world traveler in her new life.

The immortal HeLa, because of carelessness, arrogance, ignorance and lack of respect for this runaway cancer cell, has *invaded most if not all of the world's virology laboratories* including the Russian labs. The frantic HeLa is apparently unstoppable. Even pulling the stopper from a test tube of HeLa cells will spread it throughout a lab on tiny water droplets. What many scientists thought was "spontaneous transformation" of normal cells, never seen before 1951 in human cells, turned out to be simply HeLa contamination.

American scientists had developed a "unifying theory" of human cancer cells because of "certain constant characteristics" that were found no matter where the cancer came from—prostate, breast, lung, etc.—they had the same nutritional requirements and the same surface antigenic proteins. *That's because they were all HeLa cells masquerading as all the others.* Embarrassing!

HeLa spread over Europe like locusts. A lab in West Germany reported that one of their monkey cell lines was invaded and completely taken over by HeLa cells. The HeLa cells *had incorporated the viruses present in the monkey tissue* while killing off the cells. Was it a cancer virus such as SV-40? Who knows?

Nelson-Rees did some serious thinking. If the Russians were contaminated with HeLa and the Germans were contaminated with HeLa then we, who started this mess, must also be contaminated. After aR, Henrietta was from Baltimore, not Krasnoyarsk.

What he found out about "our lady friend," as he had started calling her, was extremely disturbing. He took three American cultures at random from three different labs, labeled as "breast cancer," "breast cancer" and "kidney cancer." He found that they were nothing but HeLa cells.

Next Nelson-Rees sent off a specimen to Detroit and again Dr. Peterson found the enzyme G6PD which is found only in blacks. Dr. Bassin, who had discovered the first breast cancer cell line, said that was impossible. His patient had been from the northern Mediterranean. The Centers for Disease Control must have contaminated the sample. That was certainly possible, Nelson-Rees agreed, so he asked for a fresh sample of cells from Bassin's laboratory. Again off to Detroit and again the tell-tale enzyme G6PD— the "first breast cancer cell culture" was Henrietta Lacks, the HeLa monster again.

It's disturbing to note that Bassin did his research *in the top secunty laboratwyBuilding41, of the NIH's Emergency Virus Isolation Facility.* Yet the contamination occurred. It makes you feel like you're flying m a jet with a company janitor at the controls.

Nelson-Rees found other popular cell lines to be nothing but HeLa. I won't elaborate. You get the picture. He rushed to get the word out because this was a momentous discovery. A lot of changes would have to be made. All of cancer research was involved. (They didn't know about AIDS yet.) A major scientific journal would certainly print this information about a terrible mistake so that things could be made right in the world of cancer and virology research.

First he set out to reveal the Russian "human cancer virus" hoax. The people (and scientists) would want to know that the specimens weren't anything but HeLa cells from Baltimore. He contacted the *Journal of Virology.* They were not impressed. They saw it as "a gratuitous attack on the Russians."

According to my dictionary "gratuitous" means unjustified, uncalled for, without merit. The same reviewer said, "...it really is a footnote to history and not a study with new scientific implications... I would hope... some day it would appear as a footnote." The other reviewer said if it was a footnote it would be better to put it in somebody else's journal.

After he uncovered the American part of this scandal Nelson-Rees submitted a report to the journal, Science. They rejected it although one reviewer admitted that the information was "extremely important."

Then a remarkable thing happened. Robert Bassin, the discoverer of the "first breast cancer culture" and a man of courage and integrity, reviewed Nelson-Rees' research, did a little investigating of his own and announced that a tragic mistake had occurred and that Nelson-Rees was right. That got the attention of Science and the information was published in June of 1974. Seven years later they published Nelson-Rees' final report listing over 90 different "cell lines" that were nothing but HeLa.

Like most whistle-blowers, Nelson-Rees paid a price. His funding was cut. So he quit, moved to Oakland and opened an art gallery. The brilliant detective is gone and Henrietta Lacks lives on undeterred by any nosy scientists. When it comes to grants, silence is golden.

How many honest scientists can you stuff into a phone booth? Apparently almost all of them.

Do you feel reassured by the recent National Academy of Sciences report: "There is adequate knowledge of the relevant scientific principles, as well as sufficient experience with recombinant DNA techniques to guide the safe and prudent use of such organisms outside research laboratories."?

Dr. J. Clemmensen of Denmark clearly stated her concern years before the start of the AIDS epidemic: "We are in fact establishing conditions for a possible pandemic of an oncogenic (cancer) virus variant on the scale of the influenza of 1918."9 And she concluded with this ominous note: *"It is also possible to visualize the risk of some desperate persons or nations coming into possession of some virus... so that they could threaten to spread their virus unless some requests were fulfilled."*

And to paraphrase another famous scientist: I'm not sure that scientists always do what God wants them to do.

For instance, would God approve of American scientists from the Wistar Institute in Philadelphia and the Pan American Health Organization, a branch of WHO, going into Argentina *without the knowledge of the Argentinean government* and conducting experiments on farm animals with a gene-altered rabies vaccine?[10]

9 Comp. Leuk. Res., 1973; Danish Cancer Register, 1975.
10 *Los Angeles Times*, 11/12/86.

Would God approve of giving hepatitis to dying cancer patients, in six medical centers, by the use of an experimental drug?[11]

So the burning issue confronting us would not appear to be the risk of contamination or containment at places like Elko but the *containment of scientists*—the Fifth Horseman of the Apocalypse.

The public has the mistaken conception that science is extremely precise and that the biological sciences are as exacting as, say, atomic physics. But the real world of microbiology simply isn't like that. The older microbiologists are appalled at the general carelessness and sloppiness of their younger colleagues. One scientist said that most of his colleagues were "scientific slobs." Cultures are poured down the sink and into the sewers and dangerous viruses and bacteria are treated about as casually as a jar of peanut butter from your refrigerator or a bottle of cleaning detergent from under your sink. The attitude of many of the young scientists is shockingly irresponsible, sophomoric and callous. They generally do not see beyond the walls of their own laboratories and have the attitude that if someone develops a severe infection in their lab it was their own fault and of no concern to anyone beyond that particular laboratory. It seems not to have occurred to them that they have unleashed upon the world a massive array of outlaw viruses and bacteria that will possibly change the entire ecology of the world. Chemical and radiological contamination are one thing but biological contamination is quite another matter. Chemicals and radiologicals *are not alive.*

Terrible biological accidents have happened, as we have mentioned in other chapters, and they continue to happen. One of the top laboratories in the world, and so

11 *Los Angeles Times*, 11/21/86

presumably one of the most sophisticated as far as safety measures are concerned, is the London School of Tropical Medicine and Hygiene. But in 1972 one of the workers contracted smallpox, a proper diagnosis was not made, and the worker was placed in a public hospital ward of a general hospital. The parents of a patient in an adjoining bed came to visit their daughter and sat in chairs between the beds of the two patients. Four deaths from smallpox ensued: the original patient, the two visitors and one of the attending nurses.

This is not an isolated incident. This attitude runs through all of these dangerous laboratories around the world—arrogant, irresponsible and careless.

And what happened to the smallpox virus at the hospital where the four patients died? *Did it contain itself* only to these four people? Unlikely. It's waiting somewhere. The World Health Organization celebration over the "eradication of smallpox" was premature. *Smallpox will strike again.*

June Goodfield, commenting on the critical problem of safety and the attitude of most scientists remarked that while it is far simpler and cheaper to make these biological pathogens than making an atomic bomb, "it is still unlikely that any problems will arise because of the deliberate action of some adult or even adolescent Frankenstein." Over ten years later, I wonder if Ms. Goodfield would still feel the same way in light of the experience we've had with young computer hackers who have been so clever that they have been able even to enter into the Air Force and Pentagon computer security systems?

The smallpox incident at the London School of Tropical Medicine and Hygiene was no fluke. A technician at the American Biological Warfare Center at Ft. Detrick, Maryland, once picked up an aerosol can and sprayed it around the laboratory only to find out that it was an aerosol of bubonic plage! During the last 25 years there have been 423 infections and three deaths from dangerous viruses at Ft. Detrick, Maryland, which is *maximum safey center.*[12]

At Porton Down, a maximum safety center in England, a laboratory worker died from the rare Marburg disease, a deadly African virus, when one of his protective gloves broke open and contaminated him.

Goodfield posed this question in 1977: "Can foreign DNA integrate itself in human cells and cause the kind of havoc that ultimately gives rise to cancer? ...Are the recombinant experiments likely to present to human beings in a dangerous form? Probably not."

Eleven years later we know that the answer to Goodfield's question is a very definite yes.

Dr. Sinsheimer, chairman of the biology division at California Institute of Technology, has brought up a problem hardly considered or discussed among biologists. He points out that various organisms probably have some sort of signal that prevents genetic intercourse, that is, inserting foreign genes into their genes as man is now doing. This method of control, whatever it maybe, has over eons of time prevented cabbages from inserting genes into spiders, spiders into eggplant or snakes into man, etc., etc. But what disturbed Dr. Sinsheimer is that perhaps with the splitting of DNA and inserting genes from higher to lower organisms, or lower to higher organisms, we are in a way handing over control signals to the wrong species, what Nicholas Wade calls "a sort of betrayal of state secrets at the molecular level."

There are a lot of environmentalists who worry about man disturbing the ecology. Yet, although these microbiologists are disturbing the ecology right down at the basic level, the level of the cell, one does not see Green Peace and the Sierra Club picketing Fort Detrick or Cold Spring Harbor.

---

12 Goodfield, **Playing God**, Random House, Inc,, New York, 1977. p. 116.

At the other end of the political spectrum the anti-abortion, pro-lifers, should perhaps also be picketing the laboratories at Harvard and Ft. Detrick instead of the abortion clinics. Abortion will not be a problem if there are no women left to abort. This attack on life at the very molecular level must be mounted and won, and then we can return to the political and moral issues which, without solving the basic problems, have no meaning.

Sinsheimer says that the risk of "biological chaos" is great. So these diverse political groups need to drop their differences at least temporarily and put massive pressure on state and federal governments to take action before it is too late, if it is not already too late. As one microbiologist said at the Asilomar Conference, "Nature does not need to be legislated, but playing God does." And June Goodfield adds, "The scientific profession must now face the possibility that some experiments in genetic engineering might be scientifically elegant and socially beneficial, but morally reprehensible."[13]

Science has brought us to a moral and spiritual crisis for which science has no remedy. Michael Rogers said at the Asilomar Conference, "Now that we can rewrite the genetic code, what are we going to say?" June Goodfield answers: "It is that for the first time in history, we may have the possibility of rewriting man as we know him *out of the script altogether.* It is this which fills many of us with sadness or horror. We feel that we have neither the wisdom nor the knowledge to do this." (Emphasis in the original.)

There are many brilliant and courageous scientists who are warning about the possible disaster from playing God, but who is listening? Dr. Shaw Livermore, remarking about the destruction of natural genetic barriers which separate species and thus creating a man-made evolution, said:

---

13 Ibid.

"I know of no more elemental capability, even including manipulation of nuclear forces. While it clearly would present opportunities for meeting present sources of human distress I believe that the limitations of our social capacities for directing such a capability in fulfilling human purposes will more likely bring with it a train of *awesome and possibly disastrous consequences. Decisions will be made by individuals, groups, and perhaps whole societies, that may well have unintended but irreversible effects.*"

Professor Robert Sinsheimer agrees: "Would we wish to claim the right of individual scientists to be free to create novel self-perpetuating organisms likely to spread about the planet in an uncontrolled manner for better or worse? I think not."

I suppose if you want to play God, making a toad into a prince would be as good a project as any other. But what if your end-product turned out to be half toad and half prince?

RECOMMENDED READING:

Gold, **A Conspiracy of Cells,** State University of New
       York Press, Albany, New York, 1986.
Goodfield, **Playing God,** Random House, 1977.
Kevler, **In the Name of Eugenics,** Knopf, 1985.

Chapter 6
Gene Warfare

"Another nation could be attacked surreptitiously, who could tell whether a new epidemic was natural or the result of biological warfare?"

Wall Street Journal, 4/23/84.

If scientists can now play God with germs, then generals can play Satan with these same man-made organisms. AIDS is only the opening gun, a softening up process, of a war we are losing, an arms race that is unseen and undetectable by any current spy technology.

With the advent of genetic manipulation, i.e. recombinant engineering, some most incredible and deadly viruses can now be manufactured with little difficulty. One devastating possibility would be to combine the highly contagious influenza virus with the genes of either the anthrax toxin, the botulism toxin, or the toxin from plague. If this type of designer virus were unleashed upon a population, infection of almost all of the populace would be certain, especially in the cities, and death would very quickly follow. There would be no treatment and diagnosis would be difficult. *This is not science fiction. This is today's reality.*

Some of the bio-weapons being designed by the Soviets are almost beyond human comprehension. Soviet scientists are attempting to re-combine the venom-producing genes from cobras or poisonous spiders with ordinary viruses or bacteria in such a way that once they infect the body, these organisms will produce paralytic cobra or spider neurotoxin. The Soviet literature describes these weapons as being useful in "combat or for sabotage purposes."[1]

Michael Zakharov, a former Soviet biochemist, has commented on the Soviet use of these venoms in research. He confirmed that the central Asian cobra is being used to produce one of the most powerful toxins ever known to man. He said, "If we isolate this gene—it's possible absolutely—and place it, introduce it, in the genome of a virus, what will we get? An absolute killer."

Zakharov further elucidated that perhaps the best way to deliver this paralyzing cobra venom would be to inject the cobra-producing gene into the simple flu virus. While the body was mobilizing its immune system to fight the virus, the recombinant genes would begin instructing the body to produce its own snake venom, and thus the body would poison itself.

Soviet bio-warfare scientists are also investigating the possibilities of honey bee venom, the Bulgarian viper venom and even the toxin from the puffer fish.

The *Wall Street Journal* in its series "Beyond Yellow Rain," asks, "Do these papers represent bonafide basic research by Soviet scientists, who may be looking for some new wonder drug? Or are these the 'sanitized' results of work on germ warfare? Any single one of the published Soviet research articles would not appear greatly different from basic genetic engineering research conducted in the West. Beyond doubt there are good scientific reasons to study toxins: genetically engineered drugs could perhaps kill cancer cells while not affecting healthy cells. *But the voluminous structure of the Soviet literature points to another hideous intention"* (emphasis added).

Dr. Richard Lukens, a San Diego biochemist, says, "... you see them publishing genetic engineering studies of membrane penetration and various kinds of studies you

1 Wall Street Journal, 4/23/84.

113

would expect them to do if they were in the business of improving chemical and biological warfare weapons."

The great military powers renounced chemical and biological warfare 20 years ago—and kept right on experimenting. The germ warfare experiments on Seventh Day Adventist soldiers,[2] the Tuskeegee syphilis experiments on prisoners,[3] the San Francisco Bay attack by the U.S. Army using Serratia marcescens bacteria,[4] the New York City subway germ attack[5] and many other experiments on humans, largely unknown to the victims, continue in the free world.

In Novosobirsk, the Ivanofsky Institute and other Soviet centers of biological warfare you can be sure that similar diabolical experiments on humans continue at a frantic pace.

The Soviet press, always masters of the half truth, accused the U.S. Army of having engineered the AIDS virus in the biological warfare laboratories at Fort Detrick, Maryland. This was a clever psy-war ploy which, for a while anyway, neutralized those of us who were saying essentially the same thing, that the AIDS virus was probably created through recombinant* genetic engineering and/or serial passage,** using human tissue culture cells in the top security labs at Fort Detrick. People started accusing us of spreading the communist line, not a comfortable position for dedicated anti-communists.

* Recombinant: The rearranging of genes between two or more species of animals or plants.
** Serial Passage: The growing of a virus in a series of generations of tissue cells or animals, thus adapting the virus to a new species.

---

2 "Project Whitecoat," unpublished article by William Campbell Douglass, M.D.
3 J.H. Jones, **Bad Blood**, MacMillan, NY, 1982.
4 *Common Cause Magazine*, Jan./Feb. 1988.
5 *First AIDS Report*, March/April 1988.

What the Soviet propagandists *didn't* say was that *their agents had been working in our top security biological warfare laboratories for over 20 years*. In a burst of brotherly love they were invited in by President Richard Nixon. The astounded communist scientists from Russia, the Eastern Bloc and Communist China, who had been trying to penetrate this vital security area for 40 years, quickly accepted. They have been snickering in their beakers ever since, while they prepare for our demise.

It's no secret that they are there. Dr. Carlton Gajdusek, a top official at the Fort Detrick laboratory, said in Omni magazine (March 1986): "In the facility I have a building where more good and loyal communist scientists from the USSR and mainland China work, with full passkeys to all the laboratories, than there are Americans. Even the Army's infectious disease unit is loaded with foreign workers not always friendly nationals."

You can't put it more plainly than that. Even the Greeks weren't that stupid. They didn't know the Trojan horse was full of soldiers.

When it became obvious to the Communist press that we were getting the truth out about who was running things at Fort Detrick, *they completely reversed themselves* and said it was all a mistake. Everything was just fine at Fort Detrick.

AIDS may not have been the first germ warfare attack against Americans. In the early 60's millions of unsuspecting Americans took either Salk injected polio vaccine or the live Sabin polio vaccine which was taken by mouth. *Both were laced with SV-40, a cancer-causing monkey virus*.[6] With an incubation period of 20 years, we are only now seeing the grim results of this bio-attack against Americans largely in the form of brain tumors and

---

6 *Proc. Nail. Acad Sci.*, Vol. 77, #8, pp.4861.; *Atlantic Monthly*, 2/76.

leukemia. Salk didn't like the Sabin vaccine and Sabin didn't like the Salk vaccine. I think they were both right. It is interesting to note that polio *was rapidly disappearing without a vaccine* and the vaccines probably had nothing to do with the eradication of polio.[7]

Our Soviet enemies not only instigated the AIDS epidemic through clandestine agents within our government, but *they now control,* through the World Health Organization, *the AIDS policies of the free world.*

You are probably not aware that the international AIDS prevention program of the World Health Organization (WHO) is run by the Soviets.

You don't believe it? Call WHO and ask them who is in charge in Europe. If you want to save your nickel I'll tell you. He's a Russian named Bysencho and he operates out of Copenhagen. I am not sure of the spelling of his name, but I can tell you he spells deep trouble for the west.

The Soviets control the response to AIDS of *the entire free world at many levels, including the top.* Dr. Sergei Litvinov, the coordinator of all task force work on AIDS at the World Health Organization (WHO), is a high official in the Soviet Ministry of Health. Litvinov gave out the order to our scientists and medical organizations in the western world *not* to discuss the real cause of the AIDS epidemic.

At a secret meeting between the editors of *Lancet,* the highly respected British medical publication, and a group of the leading retrovirologists of the world, it was decided not to publish any academic discussion about the possible artificial creation of the AIDS virus in a laboratory. They particularly agreed not to make any mention of world renowned biologist Isaac Farlane Burnet's published remarks that molecular biology may get out of hand like atomic physics and be used for evil purposes

7 *J. Trop. Pediat, env. Chld. Hlth.* 21,11.

and "practical applications of molecular biology to cancer research might be sinister."[8]

Other medical journals such as *Science* and *JAMA* have lockstepped with *Lancet* and put all references to the man-made origins of AIDS down the memory hole.

Did Comrade Litvinov have a little talk with the retrovirologists? They, of course, wouldn't need any encouragement from their Soviet UN bosses to attempt a little cover-up of their own heinous crime, but *Lancet*, the *British Medical Journal and the New England Journal of Medicine* are another matter. It took some powerful and sinister forces indeed to get these respected publications to cover up the crime of the millennium.

The notable exception to this appalling censorship of mass murder is Professor Harding Rains, editor of the *Journal of the Royal Society of Medicine*. Rains refers to "a conspiracy of silence" covering the allegation that AIDS was man-made. I hope Dr. Rains is watching his backside.

Dr. Zhores A. Medvedev, unlike Bysencho and Litinov, supposedly is a Russian exile. Medvedev operates out of London at the National Institute for Medical Research. He's a senior research scientist in the genetics division.

He, like Szmuness, blossomed from a poor exile into a man of power and influence. Medvedev, before he was "exiled," was head of radio-biology at a *top secret* Soviet medical research center. Since when do the Soviets exile a key scientist in the field that will be decisive in World War III—*radio-biology?*

There's a lot more about this now-British citizen and respectable scientist who continues to communicate freely with his supposed enemies in the Soviet biowarfare laboratories. We'll tell you more on page 128.

Medvedev is spreading the disinformation that AIDS is rampant in Russia due to the escape of the virus from a

---

8 Confidential information from a reliable British source.

laboratory, a sort of biological Chernobyl. This tends to divert suspicion away from Litvinov, Szmuness and the other Reds that President Nixon allowed to penetrate our biological laboratories at Fort Detrick, Maryland.

Having the Soviets "control" the spread of AIDS in the West has led to some interesting paradoxes. Our masters at the U.N. tell us that there shall be absolutely no restrictions on travel between various parts of the non-Communist world. C.E. "Chicken" Koop supports this Soviet policy of biological suicide. (Are those the instructions he received when he made his trip to Moscow where the WHO has set up its main AIDS research center?)

But, our Soviet protectors in the WHO tell us, this open policy of international travel *does not apply* to the communist bloc of nations. If you or I were to visit Moscow and tested positive for the AIDS virus, *pow*—out on the next plane. If they stay clean through *their* immigration policies and we die because of the inmigration policies imposed on us through the U.N.-controlled World "Health" Organization, who needs atomic bombs for world conquest?

Cuba, Dr. John Seale of London informs me, has a strict asylum system for the AIDS-infected. When their troops come back from "liberating" Africans, they are tested as they get off the boat. If tested positive the soldier goes directly to hell, euphemistically called a sanitarium. He can visit his family occasionally, *but only in the presence of a commissar* called a "health official" (no hanky-panky).

Unless the western world gets its act together and *closes down* the U.N., especially its genocide division called the WHO, freedom and decency will disappear from planet earth. But the problem goes much deeper. How do you close down the U.S. government laboratories such as the Centers for Disease Control (CDC), the National Institute of Health (NIH) and the Fort Detrick bio-warfare lab when the perpetrators of the crime are in control at all levels? I don't know the answer.

The Mad Scientist of the Kremlin

The most dangerous criminal in the world today does not appear on the FBI's ten Most Wanted list. The criminal to which we refer is Dr. Yuri A. Ovchinnikov.

Ovchinnikov travels freely back and forth between Russia, Europe and the United States. He is on the boards of a number of international journals of biochemistry, and doors are open to him. Ovchinnikov is the chief scientist in the Soviet Union in charge of producing modern biological weapons of incredible terror. Germ warfare is his life and he would, because of his twisted mind, feel that his life had been complete if he were able to wipe out the entire free world with one of his precious biological agents.

This ruthless man is so obsessed with power and prestige that he may very well become the head of the Soviet slave empire at some date in the not too distant future. Even the Soviets are afraid of him and recognize him as a fearful monster. However, he is *their* monster.

Professor Ovchinnikov has said, "Americans will now begin falling back in genetic engineering. We must take advantage of this to create bacteriological weapons. If we bring the Central Committee of the communist party of the Soviet Union vaccines, no one will pay attention to it. But if we bring a virus, oh, then this will be recognized by all as a great victory."

It is clear that this maniac would not hesitate to obliterate 90 percent of the human race if it enabled him to achieve his preeminence in world power. An American scientist formerly attached to the United States Embassy in Moscow describes Ovchinnikov as "one of the most dangerous men on this earth."

Like Gorbechev, Ovchinnikov is a very good actor. With his enormous thirst for power, he cannot be stopped

119

short of assassination. As one emigré Soviet biologist blurted out, "I wish someone would tell the world what that bastard is doing."

It is interesting to note the reports coming from Afghanistan where freedom fighters have reported: "Bizarre symptoms—hours of incapacitation, death so sudden it leaves victims frozen in place ...." This reference to the bodies being frozen in place sounds very much like the electromagnetic Tesla waves perfected by the Soviets which will freeze a body instantly and leave it in a state of complete preservation for months at a time.

Other bodies were found "frozen in place," but with rapid decomposition. This would be due to some type of rapid-acting virus or bacterium such as botulism, plague or anthrax tonn, causing the body to quickly rot.

If anyone doubts the intentions of the Soviets in this regard they should look at the latest edition of Military **Encyclopedia**: "Achievements in biology and related sciences (biochemistry, biophysics, molecular biology, genetics, microbiology and experimental aerobiology) have led to an increase in the effectiveness of biological agents as a means of conducting warfare. Improved methods of obtaining and using them have resulted in a qualitative re-examination of the very concept of biological weapons."

In April of 1988 the third edition of "Soviet Military Power" was published by the United States government. In this report then Secretary of Defense, Casper Weinburger, said, "There is an apparent effort on the part of the Soviets to transfer selected aspects of genetic engineering research to their biological warfare centers. For biological warfare purposes, genetic engineering could open a large number of possibilities. Normally harmless, non-disease producing organisms could be modified to become highly toxic *or produce diseases for which an opponent has no known treatment or cure.* Other agents, now considered too unstable for storage for biological warfare applications, could be changed sufficiently to be an effective agent. *In Soviet doctrine the biological weapon, is seen as a strategic weapon for the spread of infectious disease.* Many of the Soviet longand intermediate-range missile systems are technically capable of disseminating large quantities of disease agents over large areas."

The *Wall Street Journal* of April 23, 1984, commenting on Secretary Weinburger's report, said: "Another nation could be attacked surreptitiously; who could tell whether a new epidemic was natural or the result of biological warfare?" With strong evidence pointing to the AIDS epidemic as a secret bio-attack against the free world, who could, indeed.

In view of the Chernobyl disaster and the anthrax biological disaster in Russia, there is a real possibility that a biological accident could occur that would devastate both sides in this continuing war.

Even third rate nations like Libya can now create their own bio-weapons. And, as the *Wall Street Journal* reported, "...A new military organism might leap out of control of its environment, wreaking worldwide catastrophe. Even its peaceful applications have engendered fear of a genetic accident, unleashing an epidemic of some hitherto unknown disease."

Professor Joshua Letterburg said in 1970, "Scientific breakthroughs of the rather predictible kind could lead to genetically altered infective agents against which no credible defense is possible. It now appears such weapons are being developed in earnest by the Soviet Union, and that threat perhaps some day may rival even nuclear war." Indeed, Nobel Laureate Letterburg warned, biological weapons "could well become the most efficient means for removing man from the planet."

121

For the immediate future, until the communist empire has all its weapons carefully arrayed and is assured of victory, our great danger is not from attack but from a Chernobyl-like biological accident which could not only destroy us, but also the perpetrators of the crime—the Soviet microbiologists and the entire communist empire.

The Soviet record is not good. Back in the 1960s, for instance, a Russian rocket exploded on take-off and shredded a three-star army general as well as many other bystanders. Even earlier, in 1957, a nuclear accident occurred which left a radioactive wasteland in the area of Kyshtyn. Thousands of people were killed and injured and the radioactive contamination spread over a *thousand square miles* in the Techa River valley.

In the Ukraine a fertilizer plant went awry and the Dniester River was severely polluted. Drinking water became unavailable to millions of people, and tons of fish and vegetation were destroyed.

In 1983 a synthetic rubber facility exploded in Sterlitamak. This explosion was said by western experts to be of "catastrophic proportions."

Soviet Germ Warfare Backfires

Most Americans have never heard of Sverdlovsk, an industrial city of over a million people located in the Ural Mountains of Soviet Russia. But Sverdlovsk became a symbol of Russian duplicity in April of 1979 when their top secret biological warfare plant blew up, causing disease and death among thousands of people.

The explosion spread deadly anthrax spores over the city causing widespread panic. Within a week people were beginning to get extremely ill and to die and, in spite of throwing every available antibiotic at the patients and immunizing them (useless) the death toll was immense. As the rumors multiplied and the fears spread the panic reached even as far as Moscow when the news got out that the fatality rate of stricken people was over 80 percent.

Anthrax, long a popular bug for biological warfare experiments, is one of the most malignant forms of bacteria known to science. It is contained in a spore, a tough covering like that on a golf ball, and so is quite resistant to eradication. The disease is contracted primarily from the hides of sheep, cattle and other domestic animals. The organism can cause terrible weeping sores and, once in the bloodstream, death rapidly follows. It is an "aerosol spread" disease, i.e. by droplets which are inhaled. "Pulmonary anthrax" is generally fatal in spite of all efforts of modern science to save the patient. Anthrax is rarely contracted through the eating of meat, but the Soviet propagandists, after the news of the epidemic had gotten out, said the epidemic was caused by contaminated meat being sold by illegal profiteers.

All indications point to a disaster in a military biological warfare complex. Physicians in nearby towns remarked that they were never even notified about the epidemic, which would indicate that it was strictly a military problem. Many of the initial victims were members of the Soviet armed forces. The Soviet government went to extreme measures in an attempt to cover up the disaster.

Special teams of biological warfare-trained nurses and doctors were sent into the area, a number of square miles were cordoned off, and extreme measures were taken such as slaughtering of all household pets and the spraying of the tops of buildings by helicopter with powerful antiseptic solutions—hardly the type of measures that would be taken if they were dealing merely with "contaminated meat."

Some buildings at "Compound 19," the facility for manufacturing bacterial warfare agents, were sealed off and will probably remain so for 20 years.

Spy photographs revealed that there were no longer animals in the outside pens of the building. Snow on the access walks has not been shoveled since the winter of 1979-1980.

The Soviets continue to deny that there is any sort of military operation at Sverdlovsk. But American intelligence has noted the buildings, as seen from spy satellites, have special venting systems, smokestacks, refrigeration facilities, animal pens and concrete bunkers suitable for storing munitions that could be used in exploding biological bombs. It is a carefully guarded facility with double barbed wire fences and, in fact, the layout is very similar to Fort Detrick, Maryland, the center for American biological warfare activity.

It was not by mere chance that our U-2 spy plane was disabled, probably by an electro-magnetic weapon, over Sverdlovsk. Security of the air space over Sverdlovsk is extremely intense, second only to the Kamchatka peninsula with its missiles aimed at the heart of Japan. Our U-2 spy plane and pilot Gary Powers were downed when they started snooping over this biological warfare center.

It was of interest to note that, although the epidemic was blamed on "contaminated meat," a meat factory next door to the center of the accident remained open for business!

The disaster was by far the worst anthrax epidemic to have been recorded in the 20th century and perhaps the greatest one ever to be recorded. People were dying so rapidly that it became a logistical problem, as in a war, taking care of corpses. They were dumped in chloramine solution and then deposited in a common grave with the families being presented with empty coffins for burial.

In spite of this terror and chaos around the citizens of Sverdlovsk, the government announced that "nothing is happening" and told their citizens not to panic because everything was under control. The commanding general at the installation then committed suicide.

The usual apologists among the scientific community, worldwide, quickly came forward to try to cover up the obvious criminal activity of the Soviet military exposed by this disaster. The number one apologist for Soviet science in the United States, a man who is, remarkably, called upon by our government for his-opinions, is Dr. Matthew Meselson of Harvard University. Meselson is the scientist who assures Americans that the Soviet use of chemical weapons in Southeast Asia, known as "yellow rain" was nothing but bee feces! Even though Meselson came up with this incredibly stupid explanation for obvious chemical warfare in Asia he was called upon as a consultant in reviewing the situation at Sverdlovsk. Meselson bragged, "I spent many hours looking at very classified material. I disagree with the conclusions the government reached. This is all I'm allowed to say." (It was not specified by Meselson which government was not allowing him to say more.)

The report with which Meselson was disagreeing was the extensive investigation done by the U.S. Defense Intelligence Agency (DIA) which concluded: "Collectively, these events are a very strong contradiction of the Soviet position which claimed the anthrax outbreak was just a minor public health problem resulting from the sale of contaminated meat." Their analysis had been extremely thorough and proved beyond a doubt that the Soviets were indeed involved in the manufacture of biological warfare weapons and that their military installation had suffered an explosion causing the terrible epidemic.

A more clever and subtle disinformation specialist is Dr. Zhores Medvedev, who is an "expatriot" or "defector," whichever way you wish to interpret his explanations of how he left the Soviet empire. Whether he is expatriot or defector, he travels freely back and forth between London and East Germany where his brother, another scientist, is in residence. Medvedev, in a slick ploy to cover for the

Soviet military, suggested that Compound 19 was manufacturing a military vaccine against anthrax as a public health measure. American intelligence pointed out that the standard Soviet anthrax vaccine is made from a form of the bacillus which is not virulent. Being nonvirulent, it could not in anyway have caused an epidemic. Medvedev remains silent.

The party line was also followed by Dr. Vivian Wyatt of the University of Bradford, England, and by clinical microbiologist, Raymond Zilinskas. Both these gentlemen put out the refrain that "It isn't likely that the Russians would run the risk of playing around with anthrax near a vital military town" Dr. Zilinskas said, "No nation would be so stupid to locate a biological warfare facility within approachable distance to a major populated center." *All* of the Soviets' biological warfare laboratories are located near large industrial centers: Kiev, Sverdlovsk, Kalinin and Novosibirsk.

Microbiologist Zilinskas also explained that "prophylactic medication could have been quickly administered to exposed persons as public health authorities grasped the situation, and the epidemic could have been immediately stopped at that point." This reveals an obvious naivité concerning the practice of medicine. A sudden aerosol-induced anthrax epidemic would be largely uncontrollable and even if large doses of antibiotics were given, as high as 90 percent of the victims of the initial explosion would be expected to die.

One of the most effective ploys used by the apologists for the Soviets was Meselson's quoting of the testimony of Dr. Donald E. Ellis, a professor of physics and chemistry at Northwestern University. Ellis claimed that he, his wife and two small children were in the area of Sverdlovsk approximately during the time of the disaster. Ellis claimed that he saw absolutely nothing to indicate that anything at all had happened and said that "On the way to a children's camp" they passed "very close" to Compound 19. (How did Ellis, an American tourist, know about Compound 19? How would he recognize its significance even if he could read Russian signs? Even if there was no epidemic, why would he be allowed "very close" to such a facility?)

Meselson reports enthusiastically, "One of the few important certainties in this murky business is that the Soviet authorities permitted Professor Ellis and his family to enter, and, most remarkably, to re-enter the city. Although not conclusive, this does not readily fit in with the picture of an attempted cover-up of a biological warfare accident." Certainly it would be preposterous for a man, his wife and two young children to be wandering around in an area where an anthrax explosion had occurred and people are literally dying in the streets. If true, this would obviously defuse any thoughts about the epidemic having been a military biological warfare disaster or even that the epidemic occurred at all.

But in September of 1986 the Soviets panicked. There was a treaty review in Geneva and the Russians needed to put to rest, once and for all, any allegations of their working on biological weapons.

Ministry of Public Health official, Nikolay Antonov, admitted with an astonishing amount of openness, that there indeed had been an epidemic at Sverdlovsk and, he assured the scientists present, that it had been caused by "undisciplined workers" who had thrown contaminated meat into an open garbage can, after which stray dogs had spread the meat throughout many neighborhoods. Ellis, clearly, had not told the truth, but Meselson had quickly accepted Ellis, story because it was the message he wanted sent to the American people.

It is a tragedy that the United States closed down its biological warfare experimental program. Defectors and authorities on the Soviet Union have testified that the Soviets have been working on biological warfare since they took over the Soviet Union, i.e. since about 1920. We discontinued our biological research when the Biological Toxin Weapons Convention of 1972 made it "illegal for any nation to develop, produce, stockpile or otherwise acquire or retain" toxin agents.

Experts quietly agree that the technology of germ warfare makes it impossible for a treaty to be enforced and policed. The Sverdlovsk anthrax incident only emphasizes that the AIDS pandemic is almost certainly the first bio-attack against the free world, an attack which was carefully planned over a time span of about 70 years. Our enemies, if not efficient, are very patient.

The U.S. military, as in the past, is ever-ready to prove that it will never make a first strike. During the period after the second World War, due to a great deal of press propaganda, Americans developed a complex about their role in world leadership; we changed the name of our Department of War to the Department of Defense—and that is exactly what it is: defense—not offense. Bowing to the pressures of leftist scientists who are trying to prevent the United States from preparing for biological warfare Defense Department officials have said, "The policy and position of the United States is that we don't and will not possess biological or toxin weapons and that our only involvement with the subject will be for defense purposes. We are doing research in genetic engineering and related disciplines to understand what's possible. But it's for the purpose of understanding how to design a defense, not to design an offense "

This gives a clear message to the Soviets: they have nothing to fear from our biological laboratories. And the Soviet military knows that the best offense is a good offense.

The *Wall Street Journal* in its 1984 series of articles on biological warfare came to the defense of sanity and realism when they commented, "Calls to a halt of all Pentagon genetic research are clearly the worst thing we can do in the face of the Soviet threat "

The director of the U.S. arms control disarmament agency (which should be called the U.S. surrender agency), Mr. Kenneth L. Adelman, has said that U.S. officials have told Soviet officials: "We have a problem with their behavior in genetic engineering." He said that having the 1972 biological disarmament treaty in force is better than nothing "even though we believe it is being violated," but "we shouldn't let the Soviets actually off the legal hook. We should not excuse Soviet behavior one bit or lessen the amount of points we can make to people about this vile behavior on the use of chemical weapons."

What rubbish. While our agency for national suicide is tut tutting, "making points" and keeping the Soviets on an imagined "legal hook," they are well advanced in their plans to gas us to death using recombinant cobra venom bacteria.

Mr. Adelman goes on to make the brilliant remark that "arms control can't do much good, or any good, unless both sides adhere."

Richard L. Wagner, assistant to the Secretary of Defense, remarked: "We are still trying to put back together our chemical warfare and biological-defense program from years of neglect in the 1970s. We still have a long way to go, and *are now probably severely vulnerable."*

Joseph D. Douglass, Jr., an expert on biological warfare, said that "The public and civilian government officials are almost totally unprepared to respond effectively to even a crude attack by technically naive terrorists, let alone sophisticated Soviet assassins or spetsnaz troops or special undercover forces that the Soviets have infiltrated all over the world, which are to rise up at the proper moment to finish the conquering of the West. They have apparently infiltrated every nation in the free world, but to what extent is not entirely known."

The dangerous defeatist attitude of our Department of Defense is clearly evidenced by the remarks of Mr. Thomas J. Welch, a deputy assistant Secretary of Defense. Mr. Welch has said, "Retaliation by nuclear weapons is not credible in this situation (i.e. following a biological war attack). We are faced with the prospect either of defeat and horrible suffering by our people, or being driven to consider weapons we do not want to use."

It sounds as though Mr. Welch has already given up. I would recommend that he resign.

On the positive side, according to a report by the *Wall Street Journal* of September 15, 1968,, the U.S. is at last speeding development of a nerve gas bomb called Bigeye which could be delivered by carrier-based aircraft.9 Such a weapon could serve as a deterrent, presenting a potential attacker with threat of a prompt retaliation in kind.

Let's hope that it is not too late.

Surprisingly, one of the advantages of biological weapons is their portability. The uninitiated envision vast canisters of these toxic agents having to be smuggled into a country prior to their use. Unfortunately, it is much simpler. Mass production is not necessary until the agent is needed. Once a recombinant bacterium has been made with a lethal toxigen introduced, such as a scorpion or viper toxin, the cultures can be stored in a small bottle and then manufactured when the time is appropriate. Fairly unskilled but properly trained personnel can use the small cell culture to manufacture great quantities of the desired toxin or bacteria in just a few days.

Another of the negative aspects of biological warfare, from the standpoint of the aggressor, has now been

---

9 *Wall Sreet Journal*, 9/15/88.

solved Many of the bacterial agents, such as anthrax, would not be practical in their natural state because of the spores they form. The tough coat of the spore enables the anthrax bacillus to live for as long as 20 or even 30 years in a contaminated area. Naturally an invader would not want to wait 30 years to take over his newly won territory. This problem has been solved simply by making a mutant form of anthrax which does not have the tough outside protective coating. This has already been accomplished, and this new killer, Dacillus thuringiensis, is now on the shelf and ready for deployment.

One of the most momentous occurrences in science was the development of monoclonal antibodies in the mid-'70s. These antibodies, proteins that bind to cells, have been designed to fuse with cancer cells which are rapidly growing and thus will rapidly reproduce the monoclonal antibodies In this manner these antibodies can be grown outside the body in a laboratory. These hybridomas, as they are called, can produce gigantic quantities of antibodies that otherwise would be very difficult to obtain. From the bacterial warfare point of view this development was extremely important in that it enabled scientists to defeat the immune system—AIDS being the first bio-warfare example of this There will be others.

AIDS is not the type of bio-attack that our contemporary military leaders envision. They think of a bio-attack as being a sudden and dramatic flooding of the populace with some super-lethal organism that causes instant death or disability. The American people think the same way. But weapons such as AIDS are far more useful in the long run because the source is not easily detectable; there is a gradual debility of the population which is not easily explained or treated, and there is an extreme demoralizing effect psychologically, spiritually and physically. AIDS was the perfect *initial* bio-weapon to unleash on the free world A slow-acting but highly infectious agent, such as AIDS, requires the nursing time of five people for each infected person. With massive infection this will lead to bankruptcy.

Another area in which the Soviets are working is psycho-incapacitants, biological weapons which would either bring on temporary unconsciousness or agents that would cause the populace to become deranged or at least become confused for a certain period of time.

Reports from Afghanistan make it clear that the Soviets are indeed using agents of this nature. Many of the victims of this biological warfare were "frozen" in fixed positions as if they were a block of ice. There were also stories of people who have awakened after several hours with absolutely no recollection of what had happened. Some of these agents make people simply unconcerned about what is going on around them. Other agents can cause fear, rage, or simply euphoria where victims might simply come up and embrace the invader.

Many nations now have highly sophisticated gas rifles or "projecto-jets" which can expel a wet or dry agent for a distance of 600 feet to incapacitate all troops in a fairly large area. A "projecto-jet," filled with an agent called CS-1, can achieve total incapacitation of enemy troops within two seconds. Many of these agents have a very short half-life which eliminates the need to even wear protective gear. The troops only have to wait the required number of minutes or hours and then simply walk in and take over the attacked area.

A serious error in the thinking of the American military is pointed out by **Dr. Joseph Douglass** in his excellent book *America the Vulnerable.* Our military does not generally regard biological weapons as useful, because of so-called delays before onset and because of their supposed incontrollability. *This thinking is 25 years out of date.* With highly sophisticated recombinant engineering a particular biological agent can be timed to "self destruct" or to run out of potency in a designated amount of time. These weapons are now so sophisticated, as perfected by the Soviets, that they can even be designed so that the invader will know exactly when the agent will take effect, say five days from time of release.

As Dr. Douglass says, "The continued reliance on outdated 1960's scenarios by U.S. military planners is an invitation to disaster."

Very sophisticated chemical methods are now available to neutralize political leaders in the West. These agents will induce the victim to lose his sense of responsibility, cause disorientation, cause him to become extremely fatigued and unable to carry out his mission or even cause him to exhibit bizarre behavior such as exposing himself in public and becoming "drunk" and boisterous. Certain substances are now known to target specific sites in the brain. These substances are radioactively labelled and can cause permanent damage to the nervous system. They are not easily detectable and they can change a stable, dedicated, patriotic leader into anything from a fool to a homicidal maniac. This would be far more effective than simple assassination, because:

(1) It does not create a martyr and (2) It is extremely demoralizing to the leader's followers.

It would be quite feasible to infect a leader with AIDS in a hospital. It would be a very simple matter for a patient on an intravenous infusion to be injected with a massive dose of AIDS virus. This leader would slowly deteriorate, lose weight, and eventually be diagnosed as an AIDS patient, and presumably labeled as a homosexual or a drug addict. This, in my opinion, has already been accomplished with one of the major figures in the movement to expose corruption in American medicine. This particular physician was very popular, and he was the first doctor of prominence to come out strongly for quarantine of all AIDS patients.

A year after being admitted to a hospital for a few days observation, he began to lose weight. I was shocked at the emaciated appearance of this formerly robust man. A year later he was dead at age 61.

A year later I was startled to read that the Chicago Medical Society felt constrained to deny that doctors in the society had deliberately given AIDS to hospital patients!

An area of great concern is the possible poisoning of the water supplies in large urban areas. A 1967 East German military chemistry manual reported, "Great effects can be achieved in the interior, if the actions are well planned. By poisoning water supply facilities... large portions of the population can be made incapable of action for a certain period of time. Breakdowns in sensitive production areas, anxiety, uncertainty, and unpredictable actions can be the results." For many, many reasons urban water supplies are not fit to drink. But the most important reason for not drinking municipal water is the possibility of sabotage. Buy bottled water from a known supplier and never drink water from your sink unless it is from your own well.

Chlorine-resistant agents to be used in public water supplies have been developed, and it is believed that Cuba has been assigned this type of sabotage mission in the U.S. to be activated on the eve of war. Soviet-trained, Cuban Spetsnaz units have run test operations in western Europe and the United States to be certain that at the proper moment their attack will be successful. It is hard to believe that anyone would doubt that these Spetsnaz units are in place in the United States when it is realized that tens of thousands of refugees from Communist countries were allowed into the United States in the 70s and 80s, and, even today, agents from Cuba, Nicaragua, Mexico and other Spanish speaking countries flow freely across the border of northern Mexico into Texas, California, New Mexico and Arizona.

Added to this problem is the simple fact that the United States has self-destructed as far as internal security is concerned. For instance, in 1974 the Federal Bureau of Investigation had under investigation 55,000 suspects. By 1982 this number had dropped to 17– a total abnegation of the responsibility of the FBI to protect the integrity of the United States of America.

Arnaud Borchgrave testified before Congress in 1983 that the Soviet Secret Service and its Cuban division, called the DGI, operate freely in the United States and that "the DGI regards internal security in the U.S. as a joke."

One's imagination could run wild concerning Soviet involvement in many of today's interesting and unusual problems; for instance, the present epidemic of chronic fatigue syndrome, also called the Epstein-Barr syndrome. After World War I millions of people in the United States and Europe were infected with a strange disease called encephalitis lethargica or sleeping sickness. Is it possible that the present epidemic of chronic fatigue, or Epstein-Barr, is another Soviet invasion of our health through a clandestine infection such as sleeping sickness? Is this fantasy. or the ravings of paranoid right wingers? Dr. Joseph D. Douglass, author of *America the Vulnerable,* does not think so. Dr. Douglass says:

"Within the Marxist-Leninist code that governs Soviet behavior, there are no laws or morals as those terms are understood in the West. Laws and morals are derived to support the world Socialist movement, and whatever advances that movement is not only legal and moral, it is right and to be employed. This is the philosophy that needs to be clearly recognized in assessing the alarming and far-reaching implications of high tech biological warfare."

135

Even more alarming than the extensive use of biological and chemical agents in Iran and Afghanistan is the presence of such weapons in Cuba. Reliable immigrés and defectors have reported that there are at least two biological warfare facilities that have been identified in Cuba. They are so top secret that Cuban nationals *are not permitted in the plant*–they are strictly Soviet operations. As an aside, it is interesting to note that Cuban nationals are not even allowed on Cuban beaches any more; they are strictly Soviet playgrounds.

Ironically, the main bio-warfare laboratory and production center is called Jardin de Orquilles—Garden of the Orchids. The plant produces germ warfare prodUcts and toxins which are designed to be introduced into a city's water supply. Cuban army officers have bragged that these toxins could be properly placed in the Mississippi and "could contaminate a third of the United States."

The world is entering an era of cataclysmic change. Not only are we completely unprepared for these bio-warfare attacks, but we have been frozen into a state of inactivity because of left-wing and sincere but ignorant liberals clamoring for peace at any price. Even well-informed individuals in the government will acknowledge, privately, the seriousness of the situation. They are overcome with a sense of helplessness and conviction that little can be done.

Israel made a swift and decisive attack against its enemies when they saw the threat of a nuclear plant being assembled with the clear intent of destroying them. We are in a situation where we must make preemptive strikes against our enemy if we are to survive. Every bio-warfare center in Russia is known; it is also known where a major center is located in Czechoslovakia. Preemptive strikes against these facilities should be done immediately, or the war is lost.

Due, again, to misinformed idealistic liberals and a certain number of Communist agents within our own legislature, the Federal Bureau of Investigation and Central Intelligence Agency have been so emasculated that they are no longer able to monitor known subversive groups in the U.S. set up to initiate these bio-attacks.

Our best hope is local law enforcement officials, but, sadly, they are at this time very poorly trained and essentially ignorant of biological warfare.

As Dr. Douglass states in **America the Vulnerable,** "Although such drastic measures rattle the faint of heart, the prevention of biological attacks on the United States— perhaps the most bone chilling threat faced by this country—is serious business and cannot be met with halfway measures or restraint."

At present we have the ambulance-at-the-bottom-of-the-cliff mentality in which the only solution entertained is to pick up the bodies rather than go to the top of the cliff and solve the problem. If this nation does not take a more positive and pugnacious attitude we are indeed lost in the realistic world of totally amoral governments armed to the teeth with biological weapons.

Chernobyl stands as the *sine qua non* of Russian incompetence and recklessness in the area of industrial safety. Certainly the world is, to a great extent, in the hands of not only maniacs, but *incompetent* maniacs who may even destroy themselves. Our "best case" would be for the Soviets indeed to have such an accident, obliterating them, but leaving us intact—an unlikely scenario.

Through genetic alteration, the plague organism can now be made resistant to all antibiotics. The mortality rate of those infected would probably be about 99.9 percent. As antibiotics would be ineffective, the only people who would survive would be those who received photophoretic ultraviolet treatment of their blood. This excellent therapy would be available only to a selected few.

Our borders, as far as protection from infectious agents is concerned, are pathetically porous. There is absolutely no way that a terrorist could be stopped from bringing in a jar of enough Yersinia pestis or botulism toxin to wipe out an entire city.

The antibiotic era has not only put doctors to sleep, but also customs officials who are very poorly trained in communicable diseases. Immigration of officials get a very cursory training in disease recognition and are essentially useless for this purpose. The general public is also asleep on this subject and is completely indifferent to the possibility of bringing in infectious disease. Because airlines are very lax in keeping records of their customers, a plague victim could come into the United States by airline and spread it over many areas of the United States, by infecting everyone on the plane. The authorities would be unable to track down the other passengers or, by the time they did, it would be too late. With the recirculation of air in an airliner, the person with active pneumonic plague could easily infect 250 passengers. Airline managers have refused to consider the suggestion that passengers from overseas submit a card listing their itinerary. The managers say this would be too much of an infringement on the time of the flight attendants, therefore it is, they say, not feasible.

In the light of the comments of Marshall G. K. Zhukov, former defense minister of the Soviet Union, that biological weapons would be employed in future conflicts as weapons of mass destruction, it is troubling to know that we have literally no defense against these weapons. The AIDS epidemic is the first blow of a multi-focal biological attack against the free world.

Infectious diseases have not been conquered. In fact, according to Dr. Rene DuBois, the percentage of hospital beds occupied by patients suffering from infection is now as high as it was 50 years ago!

RECOMMENDED READING:

Douglass J. and Livingstone., **America the Vulnerable,** Lexington, Massachusetts, 1987.

McDermott, **The Killing Winds,** Arbor House, N.Y., 1987.

Harris, **A Higher Form of Killing,** Hill and Wang, N.Y., 1987.

U.S. House Subcommittee on Intelligence, 1980: The Sverdlovsk Incident.

Douglass, W., "AIDS As a Weapon of War," *Gung-Ho* magazine, February, 1989.

Chapter 7
AIDS, Quarantine and The Law

You will work with AIDS-infected people or else. That's the new policy of the federal government.[1]

The Office of Personnel Management (OPM) says that federal employees who refuse to work with AIDS-infected persons will be subject to "corrective action." The government, says the director of OPM, has an obligation "to show the way in *addressing the realities* of the AIDS epidemic." Director Constance Horner said there is "no medical basis for employees refusing to work with such employees."

The "reality" of the AIDS epidemic is that these people often carry tuberculosis, syphilis, hepatitis-B and many other infectious diseases. This is a perfect example of the Inverse Law of Government Action: when trying to solve a problem the government usually makes it worse.

Nation Vulnerable to Epidemics

A committee of the National Academy of Sciences says that U.S. public health efforts are in disarray, leaving the nation vulnerable to epidemics like AIDS. "We have taken our public health system for granted to the point that our guard is now down," said Richard Remington, professor of preventive medicine at the University of Iowa, chairman of the 22-member National Academy of Sciences committee.[2]

Medical authorities have gradually backed off from their original estimate that only 20 percent of AIDS-infected persons would come down with "full-blown" AIDS. (There was *never* any justification for that mislead-

---

1 AP, 4/19/88.
2 *San Francisco Sunday Examiner and Chronicle,* 9/11/88.

ing estimate.) Now, according to a report by syndicated columnist Jack Anderson, the CIA in a confidential report states that *none will survive* the AIDS virus.[3] Why do you suppose the CIA is taking such an interest in AIDS? Answer: because a sick nation cannot defend itself. Our *national security* is at stake.

Dr. James O. Mason of the Centers for Disease Control, at a talk in Huntsville, Alabama, in 1988, again put the CDC on record as opposing any serious public health approach to stopping the AIDS virus, such as universal testing and quarantine where medically necessary.

In the Soviet Union they are not so reckless with the health of their citizens or concerned about the rights of sodomists. Homosexuality gets you five years in the slammer. As there is no "confidentiality," everybody knows why you are in jail and so confinement is often a death sentence.

This antagonism against homososexuals has nothing to do with AIDS. In 7,529 homosexuals in the Soviet Union tested for AIDS not one positive case was found.[4] Dr. Wolf Szmuness, the Soviet-trained epidemiologist, didn't experiment on Russian homosexuals; only America's homosexuals got his AIDS-laced hepatitis-B vaccine.

In the general population, out of two million Soviet citizens tested, there have been *only seven AIDS-positive blood tests.* Even among 43,000 promiscuous men and women *not one case* of AIDS was discovered.

If AIDS is not a communist bio-attack against the West, then how do you explain this? AIDS is rampant in Africa, Europe, North America and South America yet virtual) absent in Russia and its satellite countries. If this plague was unexpected and accidental why did it stop at the Danube and the Berlin wall? If it came from Africa, as many have been deceived into thinking, why did it

3 *Marietta Daily Journal* (GA),12/28/87.
4 *Int. Med. News*, Vol. 21, #7.

141

spread to the United States instead of the Soviet bloc, *which has much more direct contact with Africa than we do?*

Cheating and sabotage reach their zenith in state science (the ultimate oxymoron). The Centers for Disease Control are the perfect exemplification of state science. Cheating, sabotage, tampering and suppression of data are routine. No decent scientists stay there. Of the six scientists who started the AIDS lab at CDC, five have quit.[3]

The system has gotten so bogged down in fraud and incompetence that the state of California has taken matters into its own hands and is now testing AIDS drugs which they will release when, in their judgement, the drug has promise.

Another branch of state science, the National Academy of Sciences, investigated the CDC at the request of Senator Lowell Weicker. It ended in a semi-whitewash. *The Wall Street Journal* did its own investigation and found "allegations of scientific decisions made to suit political ends" and "charges that work that was hampered might have helped thousands of people avoid exposure to AIDS." That was the Nanoxyl-9 caper. (See p. 157.)

In one act of sabotage, AIDS virus cultures were *thrown into the garbage.* (One wonders where the garbage went.) Then there was the Crimea-Congo caper. This deadly virus, which kills 40 percent of its victims, was *lost in shipment* to Maryland by the CDC. They never have found it. Maybe it's in the garbage, too.

The insane CDC guidelines on doctors with AIDS, which state that a doctor need not inform his patients of his condition, are typical. The CDC has admitted that "the regulations were a *product of compromise* between CDC and the gay community." That's politics, not science.

Paul Luciev, a geneticist at the University of California, Davis, said, "They've lost their credibility almost completely."

---

5 *Wall Street Journal*, 12/12/86.

The Augusta, Georgia, Veteran's Administration Hospital did a study to compare the effectiveness of Thorazine, a tranquilizer, with the generic form of chlorpromazine. Thorazine is the original brand name form of chlorpromazine. It costs more but, like many things, you get what you pay for.

Dr. Richard Borison, the chief of psycho-pharmacology at the Augusta V.A., conducted the study in which a group of "aggressive and violent" psychotic patients, who were well-stabilized, were switched from Thorazine brand chlorpromazine to a generic form that was cheaper.

The patients rapidly deteriorated and required up to eight times as much of the generic medication to regain control. When placed back on Thorazine they were again controlled at the old dose, a very straightforward result. This went contrary to FDA doctrine that had ruled generics to be equivalent to brand name drugs and the agency's reaction was swift and deadly to Dr. Borison's career.

The FDA ignored the information in the records, distorted the data and refused to even listen to Borison and his colleagues. They pronounced him a fraud and, without giving him an opportunity to reply, said his work was fiction. To add to the insult and embarrassment of Dr. Borison, the E;DA made their announcement at a meeting of the Generic Drug Manufacturers Association.

Several pharmaceutical companies immediately withdrew their research contracts with Borison, because "We can't work with you anymore. They're after you, on a witch hunt."6 Three FDA "inspectors" descended on his laboratory to audit his other studies for drug companies. His career was in shambles. All companies knew that he was now on the FDA hit list and therefore a nonperson.

Dr. Borison asks: "Can the FDA admit it made a mistake? Can there be other faulty investigations that we

---

6 *Med Trib.*, 12/9/87.

don't know about because the FDA has stonewalled inquiry? Can we really say the FDA is adequately protecting the public?" The answers appear to be no, yes and no.

There are four important points to be considered here:

1. If you *have* to have a drug, tell your doctor that you don't want a cheap substitute that may have been swept up from the floor of a "laboratory" in Martinique. Many AIDS drugs being brought in illegally fall into this category.

2. If this principle applies to drugs, it also applies to vaccines. Does the FDA understand that an AIDS vaccine is probably impossible and that the money could be better spent in other areas of research?

3. The government, because of corruption and inefficiency, will not solve the AIDS problem and, in fact, will make it worse.

4. We need a separation of science and state.

The story of Robert Gallo "the co-discoverer of the AIDS virus" is another case in point. Gallo claims to have discovered HTLV-I and HTLV-II. They are very different from AIDS which Gallo called HTLV-III. Now maybe he discovered I and II and maybe he didn't, but he most emphatically did not discover AIDS.

Dr. Luc Montagnier announced the discovery of the AIDS virus at the Pasteur Institute in Paris in May, 1983. The French scientists actually saw the virus for the first time and photographed it on February 4, 1983.

These dates are important because Gallo was to claim a year later that he discovered the AIDS virus and that it was obviously just a variant of his HTLV viruses. They knew it was AIDS all the time, Gallo said. They just hadn't gotten around to photographing it or bothering to tell anybody about it.

Can you imagine that? You've got the medical discovery of the century in your hot little hands and you don't photograph it or announce it for *15 months?* Then when you do publish your momentous discovery the photographs turn out to be the ones the French took a year before? Gallo said that was a mistake. The lab technician mistook "LAV" on the specimen to be the patient's initials. What kind of lab tech, working in the AIDS field, wouldn't know that LAV stands for Lymphadenopathy Associated Virus— AIDS? Come on, Robert, what was the patient's name, Louise Augustus Veritas?

One of the co-authors of the article containing the French photographs quickly denied any responsibility. He said don't hang this on me, the article was Gallo's idea. He has since fled to a European lab.

Remember that Dr. Robert Gallo, Max Essex of Harvard and the other virologists in the driver's seat of the National Cancer Institute work with and for the government. In that position they have tremendous power to blow smoke, confuse, delay, deny and do just about anything else to turn things their way and bury competitors. That's government science, and the way Dr. Montagnier's monumental discovery was buried is typical.

Montagnier submitted his article to the journal, Science. Gallo and Essex, knowing that the article was to be published and, having read it, instead of supporting Montagnier submitted articles for the same issue on AIDS touting the "link" of AIDS to Gallo's HTLV viruses.

AIDS is not an HTLV virus but the articles accomplished their purpose. The journal itself ignored the great medical breakthrough of the French and focused on the inaccurate work of the scientists they are beholden to. Gallo and Essex were quoted extensively. With the AIDS virus discovery right in their own magazine, they gave it one sentence of comment. The discovery of the AIDS vi-

145

rus went unnoticed and the greatest biological killer in the history of the world had another year to spread among the world's population—unhindered.

The real co-discoverer of the AIDS virus is Dr. Abraham Karpas of Cambridge University. He described a virus from his AIDS patients but he said it was unrelated to HTLV. Because he wasn't on the Gallo HTLV bandwagon, he said he had difficulty getting his work published. His research went to the "Gallos," so to speak.

Karpas is a little bitter as you might expect. "Gallo's preoccupation with HTLV as the cause of AIDS," he said, "led many people in the wrong direction at a critical stage in AIDS research. A full year was wasted. In that time many lives could have been saved, many infections could have been prevented."

Gallo didn't have the AIDS virus but he sure did have the press. Through the *Wall Street Journal, the Washington Post* and other major papers he announced on April 19, 1984, that he had found an HTLV "variant" which was probably AIDS. Four days later, *and a year after the actual discovery by the French,* the Department of Health and Human Services announced that Gallo and Company had "discovered" the AIDS virus! More government science.

The HTLV-AIDS fiasco isn't Gallo's first excursion into weird science. In 1975 he announced in a paper that he had discovered a new human virus that was involved in human leukemia. Other researchers proved that his new virus was a soup composed of three ape viruses: gibbon, baboon and a simian sarcoma. Gallo admitted that "It was bizarre." It wasn't just bizarre. It was very bad science.

Dr. Robert Gallo, because his public relations ability more than makes up for his lack of scientific consistency, will probably win a Nobel prize as the "co-discoverer of the AIDS virus." Dr. Luc Montagnier had better watch out or he'll get elbowed right out of the picture. As for Cambridge's Dr. Karpas, he'll be lucky to get a ticket to the ceremony.

For many Americans, science has replaced religion as the source of truth and values. So we have a state religion called Science, and Evolution is Book I. In the beginning there was Atom, not Adam.

The state supports its religion through grants of tens of millions of dollars to the right apostles. People like Gallo control this money and therefore determine what is good science and what is bad science. Good science is that which doesn't disturb the status quo in research or business. Nothing good can come of it.

If you don't think business controls science then you are naive in the extreme. Dr. Gallo's insistence that his HTLV-III was the AIDS virus had momentous economic effects. Backed by his boss, the Department of Health and Human Services, it was announced to the American press that Dr. Robert Gallo had discovered the AIDS virus—a year after the French had done so. Genetically, through a technique called restriction mapping, *it was proven beyond a doubt that Gallo's "discovery" was simply the AIDS virus out of a test tube supplied to him by the scientists of the Pasteur Institute in Pans.*[7]

Everyone knew that billions were to be made by the group that first produced a laboratory test for AIDS. But first the organism had to be identified. You can't test for something until you know what you are testing for. The end result of Dr. Gallo's publicity ploy, in collusion with other health bureaucrats of the U.S. government, was *to block the French from getting a US. patent on an AIDS test.*

Pasteur applied for its first patent in Britain in September, 1983. Gallo applied on April 23, 1984, seven months later. The U.S. government awarded a patent to Gallo a

---

7 *New Scientist*, 2/12/87.

year later and the French were left waiting. As profits soared into the hundreds of millions of dollars, the French sued—and won.

There is a pharmaceutical, called ribavirin, that has a low toxicity, definitely helps patients in the early stages of AIDS, has been used by thousands of people and doesn't require blood transfusions to keep the drug from killing the patient. It is so non-toxic that it has been used in newborn infants without any serious side effects. *The head of FDA, D,: Frank Young has admitted that the drug is effective in the treatment of certain neonatal illnesses.* Yet AIDS patients have to go to Mexico, and pay through the nose, to buy this California produced drug.

In the face of his own remarks to the contrary, *Dr. Young says that ribavirin is too toxic* and so he has held up its release.

Why is Commissioner Young lying about this drug? There are several possible explanations, all very ugly. Some have suggested that the FDA is *waiting for the majority of the homosexuals to die off* before releasing ribavirin. AZT is a killer drug offering *absolutely no hope* to the AIDS sufferer. So this may not be as far-fetched as you think. You wouldn't think any decent American would want to withhold a drug that could relieve suffering but money and mercy don't seem to mix.

The other explanation is greed. *ICN Pharmaceuticals, Inc.,* the manufacturer of ribavirin ("Virazole"), is a small company with little political influence. It's president, Milan Panic, seems to have difficulty dealing u~th bureaucrats. (You can understand that.) He can't understand why a drug that will probably have many uses beyond the treatment of early AIDS *(hepatitis, flu, herpes),* is far less toxic than all of the cancer drugs on the market and has been thoroughly tested on hundreds of people, should not be released.

The FDA did a first class hatchet job on Panic, his company, and the scientists who did the research for ICN. The FDA hatchet persons, Drs. Moledina and Cooper, misled Congressional investigators with *faulty statistics that made ribavirin appear to be killing rather than helping the AIDS patients.*

The data that the FDA had in hand from the company, but did not reveal to the committee, proved the opposite, i.e., the death rate among ribavirin users (1.3 percent) was considerably lower than the non-users (11.3 percent).

Based on the incomplete statistics that they revealed, Dr. Moledina was asked if it was true that "the more of this stuff you took, the better your chances were of dying."

Moledina replied, "That's what it seems like (but) I cannot at this time make that conclusion." In other words, that's what we want you to assume although we haven't proven it.

Dr. Cooper added that the only definite conclusion she could make was that some of the patients died!

Drs. Moledina and Cooper are a couple of kids fresh out of school. They are in their late 20's and yet are able to overrule the opinions of many seasoned, expert men of science simply because they are designated experts by a federal regulatory agency.

Moledina and Cooper hang out a lot at the National Institute of Health, the payola group we mentioned a few paragraphs back. I'm sure they are having a wonderful learning experience but do you think kids who still get off on Bruce Springsteen records should control the destiny of cancer and AIDS research in this country? Should their opinion be accepted *over four experienced researchers and four world-class statistical experts* who all agreed that the studies proved that ribavirin was effective?

The FDA has now agreed to "further testing" of ribavirin—another stall tactic. They have also stated privately that they are "no longer concerned about the safety

149

of ribavirin." But they have done nothing publicly to correct the slander and discredit they brought to ICN Pharmaceuticals and its researchers which caused many patients and doctors to abandon the drug out of fear of doing harm when it was actually helping them.* How many lives were shortened because of FDA lying and duplicity?

The reason for all this prevarication is very simple. The killer drug AZT was developed by the National Institute of Health (NIH), a tax-supported medical government bureaucracy. NIH licensed AZT to the Burroughs-Welcome pharmaceutical company very quickly and, according to many, without proper testing. Burroughs-Welcome pays royalties back to NIH just as if the National Institute of Health was a private company.

Why does a corporation pay "royalties" to a government body? Where does the money go? Why did Burroughs-Welcome get the license? Were there bids by other pharmaceutical companies? NIH has been touting AZT almost as much as Burroughs-Welcome. Do you suppose they do that out of altruism?

Now the NIH has come out with Son of AZT called DDC (dideoxycytidine). The NIH in its lust for power and glory is in collusion with the FDA to keep Virazole off the market in order to give DDC the lion's share of the AIDS market.

Big business is not our problem. It's big government which encourages corruption in business and in government-controlled science. This leads to merciless exploitation of the American people.

Dr. Irwin Bross is giving up on state science. He wrote a brilliant letter to the *American Journal of Epidemiology*[8] in

---

* For a detailed analysis of the ribavirin testimony write to: Mr. Dennis Roth, 905-16th Street NW, Washington, D.C. 20006. Enclose $2.00 for postage and handling.

8 *Amer. J. Epidem.*, Vol. 120, #1, p.167.

which he stated that the federal government has become the adversary of its own citizens in litigation concerning the health effects due to the misuse of technologies. "Since 1955," Bross said, "official science has been steadily replacing genuine science in many areas... and the process by which technical journals became house organs of official science was so gradual that few realize what has happened."

Dr. Bross condemns the scientific journals for being more concerned with "protecting their government grants than with protecting the public health" and he concludes: "Perhaps the only way for genuine science to survive is to adopt the rules used for religion: a separation of Science and State just as the constitution requires separation of Church and State."

AIDS Doubletalk

There are some strange contradictions going on among public health officials concerning AIDS. Dr. Otis R. Bowen, then Secretary of Health and Human services, warned that AIDS was "rapidly spreading" into the general population and would make the Black Death "pale by comparison"

Only six months later he recanted and stated that his earlier prediction "had been alarmist."

Why would such an important public health official completely reverse himself in only six months? American Health magazine[9] comments that "no one knows how widespread HIV infection really is in America, because conclusive studies haven't been done... forecasts remain only educated guesses."

One can't help but wonder if Dr. Bowen wasn't ordered to change his opinion on the spread of AIDS.

---

9 *American Health,* June, 1988.

The Chimp Killers of the NIH

The National Institute of Health is attempting to run around the international agreements concerning the use of chimpanzees for use in AIDS research.

In 1978 the chimpanzee census revealed that chimp populations are extinct or greatly depleted across much of their traditional African range. In West Africa, for instance, the census has dropped from a million to about seventeen thousand. The director of the NIH, James Wyngaarden, confirmed in an interview that the agency is considering doing AIDS research projects in Africa and the Soviet Union, because U.S. law bans importation of chimpanzees. The Associated Press, by obtaining confidential minutes of the NIH, discovered that they were planning to identify target areas in Africa where the few remaining chimpanzees could be exploited and used for AIDS research.

It's interesting to note that one of the possible sites for research in Africa would be Liberia at a lab operated by the New York City blood bank—the people who brought AIDS to America's homosexuals.

Dr. Jane Goodall, a world authority on chimpanzees and gorillas, stated that these new chimpanzee roundups, during which hunters often kill adults in order to get at the young, "would not only have a devastating effect on chimpanzees, but would bring them to extinction." *An average of 10 mothers and babies are killed for every infant chimp successful) exported.*

An American primatologist, Dr. Geza Teleki, said, "The NIH clearly intends to continue being an accomplice in driving the species to extinction beyond the view of the American public."

Because chimpanzees are so closely related to humans (less than one percent genetic variation), chimpanzees are essential for AIDS research. However, many authorities have pointed out that not enough is done to encourage breeding in captivity which could supply enough chimpanzees if this avenue were pursued. Marc Girard of the Pasteur Institute said, "Going to Africa is no solution. We must breed more, better use those we have and find alternatives."[10]

Operation Fruitcake

The Post Office is becoming a dangerous place to work. In Kansas City the Post Office has issued gloves, aprons, masks and iron tongs to postal workers.

Blood and urine stained mail has been coming through Kansas City and the people are upset about it. The blood and urine samples, mailed from all over the United States, are destined for a lab near Kansas City. Officials are singing the usual song—infection is "unlikely." Broken glass and infected blood sounds "likely," not unlikely.

According to the *Wall Street Journal* there is a suspicion that certain genetically engineered viruses, more deadly than natural ones, maybe included in the Army's mail order business.[11] "Certain genetically engineered viruses," could include T-cell leukemia virus, brain tumor virus (SV-40) and HIV—AIDS.

The Dugway Proving Grounds is in Utah, 70 miles from the nearest city. It's a laboratory for testing deadly viruses essential to counter the Soviet threat in biological warfare. The Army is advising an increasingly skittish public that the safeguards being set up there are "virtually foolproof"[12] The colonels used 200 pages to describe how safe the lab will be. But on the 201st page they give you the Laurel and Hardy punch line: organisms such as

---

10 *Times-Union*, Warsaw, Indiana, 6/9188.
11 *Wall Street Journal*, 4/5/88.
12 Ibid.

anthrax and encephalitis will get to the lab the way your Aunt Hattie sends her fruitcake—by U.S. mail. "They're going to wrap them up and drop them in a mailbox? That's incredible," says Dr. Richard P. Novisk, director of the Public Health Research Institute.

CDC — The Tip of the Iceberg

A scientist once said, "There are two kinds of research in the pharmaceutical industry, fraud and gross fraud." The motivating factors in the pharmaceutical industry for fraud are fame, power and money. In the U.S. Centers for Disease Control (CDC) it's fame, power, and eventually money. (After you leave and join the opposition in the food or drug industry.)

Sometimes you can kill people simply by withholding vital information. Look what happened at the Bay of Pigs. Life's tough enough without having people pull the rug out from under you.

Do you think people at the CDC would withhold vital information about a preventive for AIDS that is simple, cheap and extremely effective? Would they do a cruel thing like this because "curing" has fantastic rewards (if you are first) and "preventing" doesn't?

You are aghast at the thought. Science doesn't work that way. Science is impartial, altruistic, self-correcting, noble, honest, exacting, unemotional, and accurate. Science is none of the above and if you think it is then you are suffering from a terminal case of sciencephilia, a disease common to atheists, fools, and many college graduates.

In August, 1986, the Associated Press reported a typical case of scientific fraud at the national Centers for Disease Control It was revealed that "tens of thousands had become unnecessarily infected with the deadly AIDS virus because of suppression of data by the CDC." Researchers at the CDC had discovered that simple spermicide cream (Nanoxyl-9), available at any drug store, will kill the AIDS virus in 60 seconds. This information was not released to the public.

But this CDC fiasco is only the tip of the iceberg. A few months later another scandal broke at a major university. A researcher was discovered to have falsified his work. He admitted: "I was disappointed in the results. I just couldn't stand it." Then he fled to his home country of Syria never to be heard from again.

California Capers

It is said, "As goes California so goes the nation." California law to protect AIDS patients has gone so far as to completely emasculate any effective disease-containment by public health authorities and doctors.

In California it is now a criminal offense for a doctor to reveal the HIV status of one of his patients. In September of 1987 a law was passed which allows the doctor to disclose test results to the "spouse" of the patient but no one else.* If a man has AIDS and his partner is another man does this classify as a "spouse"? If a woman has AIDS and her partner is another woman does that classify as a "spouse"? Even the Public Health Department itself cannot be notified of the AIDS positive status of the patient!

As pointed out by Dr. William T. O'Connor in his monograph: "AIDS The Alarming Reality," this leaves the people of the state of California completely unprotected from the deadly disease. He says that health authorities cannot:

1. Collect valuable data about the disease.
2. Find out who an infected individual has had sex with.
3. Stop irresponsible behavior by carriers.

---

* After January, 1989, California doctors will be allowed to inform other medical personnel as well as "sexual partners" about HIV exposure but not the source of that exposure! (*Wall Street Journal*, 11/2/88.)

4. Even test a confirmed rapist for AIDS.
5. Test people who intentionally attempt to transmit the disease such as by biting a police officer.
6. Inform people who are tested anonymously that they have the disease.

In other words the law has been turned against doctors sincerely trying to protect the public in order to protect the "rights" of a largely irresponsible segment of society. In the name of decency and medical ethics, many doctors will break this law by anonymously informing those threatened.

In Texas and California, and many other states, prostitutes, both male and female, are allowed to continue to ply their trade even though they are AIDS-infected. It is ironic that prostitution, which is illegal in every state but one, is protected from time-honored public health regulations. Nothing will stop prostitutes from plying their trade except severely repressive measures. These actions should include incarceration, castration, and even execution if this is what is required to save our civilization.

Dr. O'Connor says, "... recall that there is no foreseeable cure or vaccine, the limits of transmission have not been determined as yet..." and these infected people are most certainly rapidly spreading the disease. Dr. O'Connor added, "As long as these irresponsible people are allowed to freely circulate through our society, they will continue to spread the disease with nothing to stop them, not the Public Health Department, not the physicians and, in most cases, not even their own conscience."[13]

Governor Deuknejian of California said, in defending his support of the defeated AIDS reporting bill: "I came to the conclusion that because the disease continues to spread, that if you believe that life is sacred, then I think

---

13 O'Connor, *AIDS: The Alarming Reality*, POB 808, Vacaville
   CA 95696.

that society has to do everything that it possibly can do to protect the lives of innocent people."[14]

The bill was opposed by most of the professional medical organizations including the California Medical Association and the California Nurses Association. The opposition brought out their big gun, Surgeon General C. E. Koop, to educate the people of California. The usual arguments, "discouraging research," "driving the infected underground," "violation of the right to privacy," "loss of job," etc., were invoked, and the measure was, predictably, defeated.

Proposition 102, clearly a backlash against homosexuals, would have required doctors and blood banks to report to state health officials anyone who tests positive for the AIDS virus. This return to sanity and good science was supported by a large minority of California voters although it was defeated. Dr. Koop said, "There's no one in public health who supports this measure. It is contrary to every principle of public health I know."

In response to this outlandish statement, promoters of the amendment called for the resignation of Dr. Koop. Paul Nero, a spokesman for Representative Dannemeyer of California, said that Koop's anti-102 comments "were to be expected" since the Surgeon General has consistently opposed efforts to make AIDS-reporting a federal law.

AIDS Testing

Dr. Neal Schram, a member of the Los Angeles County Medical Association AIDS Committee, said that syphilis was a good example of why testing and identification doesn't work. He said that the spread of syphilis was not curtailed until a cure was found thus implying that identification and quarantine was useless. But then he said

---

14 *San Francisco Examiner*, 11/5/88.

later in his comments that syphilis is now out of control in Los Angeles county.

If syphilis is now out of control, and we have an effective cure, this can only mean that it is out of control because public health authorities have become lax in their testing and identification of this disease. Even if we were to have a cure available tomorrow, testing and identification of AIDS-infected people would be absolutely essential if we are to stop this epidemic. It's no wonder that the people have lost confidence in public health officials and doctors when they come up with such insupportable arguments against testing and quarantine.

Is the State Government Part of the Problem?

The state of New York is quietly channeling funds into the homosexual movement in New York City. $100,000 has been given to several homosexual activist groups by the New York State Council for the Arts. The council is funding a photographic exhibition and lecture series designed to encourage transvestism.[15] The state is also funding a homosexual magazine for lesbians. With only 534 paid subscribers, the $6,000 grant to *Conditions* magazine is costing N.Y. taxpayers $11.23 per subscriber copy while subscribers pay $8.95. Seems to me that $20.18 is a lot for a dirty magazine even in New York.

By 1991, according to a *Medical Tribune* report, as many as 10,000 full-time hospital beds will be needed every day in New York City for the in-patient care of persons with AIDS. *One in seven* prisoners in the New York City jails now tests positive for AIDS. About 70 percent of all New York state's prisoners come from New York City—the AIDS capital of the nation.[16]

The CDC has advised hospitals that extreme caution should be exercised around AIDS patients. Masks and

15 *N.Y. Post*, 3/16/88.
16 Op. Cit., 3/24/88.

gloves should be worn; clean with bleach, etc. Children are being forced to go to school with AIDS patients even if they have a cough or runny nose but no one has suggested masks and gloves for *them*.

The state of New York has purchased 1.5 million pairs of disposable gloves for teachers and public school employees. They are for "giving assistance to a person who is bleeding" and "cleaning up blood or other bodily wastes." Wouldn't it be safer to *remove the infected people* from the schools? Don't well children and teachers have a "civil right" to protection from a deadly disease?

The New York Health Commissioner, Dr. Stephen C. Joseph, estimates that there are "up to 1,000 infected school children in the school system."17 But, of course, these AIDS-infected children are "no danger to themselves or others." Then why is he issuing *five pairs of disposable gloves to every teacher and school staff member?* Along with disposable gloves we now have disposable children.

Reagan's AIDS Commission In Disarray

The executive director of the AIDS commission quit in September, 1987. The chairman, Dr. Eugene Mayberry, quit October 7 without explanation. The vice chairman, Dr. W.A. Myers, quit the same day. A power struggle had developed between chairman Mayberry and Dr. W.B. Walsh, another committee member. The administration failed to back up the chairman.

The members, who know little about AIDS and one of whom is a homosexual, can't even agree on the purpose of the commission. You know the definition of a camel: a greyhound designed by a committee.

Then the AIDS commission was taken over by Admiral James Watkins, who turned it into a one-man crusade

---

17 *Spotlight*, 11/2/87.

for civil rights. Watkin's proposals, which have become law, tranfer much of the cost of caring for AIDS patients from the government to private business. This will eventually bankrupt the private insurance industry and lead us further down the road to a socialist police state.

The history of reporting of infectious disease in England reveals many parallels with the arguments given today against identification of the AIDS-infected. Tuberculosis in England was increased by the general unwillingness of doctors to report tuberculosis to public health officials. Some considered it an "administrative nuisance," and others felt a reluctance to lose the patient to the tuberculosis authorities. Some doctors did not report out of a sense of compassion: "It is not uncommon for a patient with definite early symptoms of tuberculosis to escape notification because the physician wishes to avoid the effect of such an action on the general life and future of the individual."[18] And with echoes of the AIDS epidemic, many physicians objected to reporting because of the handicap to individuals of not being able to get life insurance.[19] Also reminiscent of our present AIDS epidemic, patients were often reluctant to report their initial infection to a doctor. There was "the fear and dread with which the disease is held by the lay person."[20]

It was thought that notification would, as today, jeopardize employment opportunities for the infected and, as Bulstrode pointed out: "No human beings...are anxious to advertise the fact that they are suffering from a malady which the public is beginning to believe is, as regards infectivity, on a par with smallpox .... "[21]

---

18 *Tubercle*, 20,1939.
19 Bryder, **Below the Magic Moantain,** Oxford University Press, 1988, p. 107.
20 Ibid.
21 The Bulstrode Report, late 19th Century.

In reply to this Sir John Robertson said: "Compulsory notification does not mean public identification."[22]

In spite of massive tuberculin "immunization," various efforts to "uplift" the poor morally, and the presence of 97 sanitoria, 83 isolation hospitals and 79 voluntary institutions, the death rate from tuberculosis in England was not affected one whit. As with polio in the 20th century, the death rate from TB had been steadily falling since 1850 without any definitive treatment. With the introduction of the chemotherapeutic anti-tuberculosis drugs, the death rate from tuberculosis gradually dropped from a high of 380 cases per 100,000 in 1850 to about 30 cases per 100,000 by 1950. But in spite of fifty years of anti-tuberculosis chemotherapy, tuberculosis is now making a rapid comeback throughout the world. Will polio, smallpox, yellow fever and plague do the same?

The only thing that even *partially* worked was quarantine, and quarantine is the only thing that will work today.

Compulsory notification of tuberculosis was introduced in 1913 which required all tuberculosis cases to be reported to medical officers who would then follow up to prevent further spread. Some doctors also argued that notification interfered with the confidential doctor-patient relationship. Today that argument seems to be turned around in that doctors are saying that it's unethical for them not to report AIDS cases to the proper authorities and to the families of the infected persons.

It is interesting that "Article 16" of the British regulations stated, "The medical officer has no power to enforce any enactment which renders the person, or any other persons, liable to any restriction, prohibition, or disability affecting himself or his employment on the grounds of suffering from tuberculosis." If carried out to the letter,

---

22 Ibid.

this regulation would have prevented quarantine of anybody and, in fact, it was ignored.

Bryder said: "There was a fear and dread with which the disease is held by the lay person, a sense of fatalism, social stigma attached to the disease, the prospect of supervision and threatened invasion of his or her home by the authorities, and finally and possibly most important of all, the fear of losing his job as a result of being discovered to be tuberculous and the financial consequences for the patient and family which this entailed."[23] Just change the word "tuberculosis" to "AIDS-infected" and you have entered a time machine—and landed in the late 20th century.

Human attitudes on something as important as personal liberty (and responsibility) have not changed. We are again facing the same fear, dread, loss of liberty and inevitable death with this disease as the world did in the 19th century from tuberculosis. We should be at least as intelligent and realistic as our brethren of the late 19th century and impose quarantine with a disease which is far more deadly than tuberculosis, impossible to treat effectively and, even in this late 20th century era, unclear as to its means of transmission.

Dr. Robert Koch, in his Nobel lecture of 1906, pointed out the dramatic decline in leprosy which occurred as a result of isolation of lepromatous patients.

Dr. Theodore D. Acland wrote in 1907:"As long as the only refuge for a man who is dying of tuberculosis is the workhouse infirmary there cannot fail to be much damage done by people refusing to go into the infirmary, and infecting their families by staying at home."

Dr. H.H. Thomson, a tuberculosis specialist, said in 1912 that it was remarkable, after the amazing results of

---

23 15th Annual Report Ministry of Health, 1933-34, Cmd.
    6446, 69.

segregation on the number of cases of leprosy, that steps were not taken to isolate tuberculosis patients sooner.

Except for some improvement in nutrition, quarantine was probably the only thing the doctors of the late nineteenth and early twentieth centuries did that had any effect whatsoever on the tuberculosis epidemic. So quarantine, although it may not appear humane, may in the long run be the most humane thing that we could do, as well as being sensible public health policy.

In a recent poll 28 percent of physicians queried felt that AIDS patients should be quarantined.[24] If quarantine is not instituted before critical mass is reached, and such a large percentage of people are AIDS-positive that no political action is possible, then the uninfected will quarantine *themselves* in an attempt to avoid the holocaust. It is not difficult to envisage small groups of people huddled together in remote areas and "circling the wagons" against the outside world. In a nation where civil rights are more revered than civil responsibility, this may be the only means the uninfected part of the population has to protect itself from persons with AIDS. If strong action is not taken soon there is little doubt that the AIDS virus will permeate the entire population with the consequent death of hundreds of millions.

Many nations are being realistic and taking strong measures to protect their citizens. Sweden puts all AIDS patients on an island. Cuba has set up quarantine centers for the AIDS-infected. The Soviet Union, Korea, China, Japan and many others are far ahead of the United States in preparing for this global plague.

Although this nation is drenched in "technology," the only form of technology we have at the present that has

---

24 MD magazine, January, 1987.

any hope of succeeding in stemming the tide of AIDS is the technology of quarantine. If we are not to go the way of the Mayas and the Incas, strong quarantine measures must be instituted immediately.

Quarantine is a technology that works. With an incurable disease it is the only technology that works. If we do not employ it soon, the war is over. Modern science may, in the long run, save us. But we simply must not abandon a proven form of preventive medicine or we will not be able to buy the time needed for future technology to stem the tide.

RECOMMENDED READING:

O'Connor, *AIDS: The Alarming Reality,* P.O. Box 808, Vacaville, CA 95696.

Bryder, **Below the Magic Mountain,** Oxford, 1988.

Chapter 8
Heterosexuals, AIDS and Casual Contact

The "sex experts," Masters and Johnson, generated considerable controversy in early 1988 with their book, Crisis: **Heterosexual Behavior in the Age of AIDS.** The message of the book is that heterosexuals are indeed catching AIDS and that the degree of infection has been hidden from the American people. Masters and Johnson were immediately attacked by practically everyone. It was unique to see writers on the right, such as Patrick Buchanan, joining the leftist media and the government in attempting to debunk the findings of Masters and Johnson.

It is curious to see conservative-writers, who are generally realistic, grasping at any reports or facts that will enable them to deny the threat of the AIDS epidemic. This peculiar attitude is probably rooted in a fear of increased government control over our lives, even possibly including martial law, as an answer to the AIDS epidemic. This attitude is certainly understandable, and there is no doubt that this is a real possibility. However, ignoring the threat of the AIDS epidemic will not in any way help solve the problem but, in the long run, will only make it worse.

Anyone who reads the Masters and Johnson book cannot help but be impressed with the statistics they present and the opinions derived therefrom.

It is undoubtedly true that most of the people who criticize the book have not even read it and are taking the Opinions of others, or merely giving out opinions based on what they hope to be true. These critics should at least read chapter 3 of the book before passing judgement and, after having read this chapter, most of the honest critics will have to admit that Masters and Johnson have a point.

Their most shocking finding, in fact a staggering revelation, was that the incidence of AIDS among "highly active" adults is astronomically high. They defined "highly active" adults as having more than six sexual partners a year for the past five years, a very large group of Americans. *In the study group they found an AIDS-prevalence rate of five percent among the men and seven percent among the women.*

This means that for a person with six or more sexual partners per year the risk of catching AIDS is 24 times as great as for a monogamous person. If a person has 12 partners per year, his likelihood of catching AIDS is 52 times as great. Put in realistic terms, if Masters and Johnson's figures are correct, *one in eight of the young people cruising the singles ' bars is infected with AIDS.*

As stunning as the above findings are, perhaps even more unsettling is their finding that "High risk sexual behavior" made no significant difference in the rate of infection. Therefore the warnings of the Surgeon General on condoms and "safe sex" are probably doing more harm than good because of giving these young people a false sense of security. Masters and Johnson estimate that there are over three million AIDS-infected individuals in our population who not only don't know they are infected but don't believe, because of inappropriate government propaganda, that they have any possibility of being infected.

The raw nerve touched by Masters and Johnson concerning quarantine was no doubt a major factor in producing animosity among government officials and liberal-thinking Americans. The authors bluntly state, "The sexual revolution is not dead, it's just that some of the soldiers are dying."

The reactions of government officials, such as Dr. C. Everitt Koop and Dr. Robert Windom were instant and vicious.

The authors were hit with the same epithets that others have received for pointing out the terrible truth: "Irresponsible," "scare tactics," "needlessly alarming," "a very serious setback in AIDS education," "senseless hysteria," and, of course, they are accused of "commercializing on the fear of AIDS."

Dr. Windom, assistant secretary for HEW, stated flatly, "AIDS is not exploding into the heterosexual community."

One wonders how Dr. Windom would explain this report from the *Journal of the American Medical Association (JAMA): Eight percent of the husbands and eight percent of the wives of spouses infected by contaminated transfusions became infected with the AIDS virus over a period of two to three years."*[1]

Also from *JAMA:* 76 percent of husbands and 50 percent of wives were infected through sexual contact with their infected spouses.[2]

Three percent of women of child-bearing age in New York City have been found to be infected with the AIDS virus and five percent of people in the emergency ward at Baltimore's Johns Hopkins University Hospital are infected. As many of the women in the New York City report were pregnant, we can assume that they are heterosexuals.

A Hudson Institute report reveals that as high as 25 percent of symptom-free men carrying the AIDS virus will test negative on conventional antibody tests. *Nine percent of people with no known exposure to AIDS tested negative on a conventional probe who were nonetheless found to be carrying the virus.* The Hudson Institute reports: "There are two main implications of these findings. One obviously is that a negative antibody test does not necessarily signify the absence of HIV infection... This result makes the serial prevalence surveys conducted to date almost useless ...."

1 *Journal of the American Medical Association,* 1/1/88.
2 Op. Cit., 2/6/87.

Another article from the *Journal of the American Medical Association* reported that the number of heterosexual AIDS cases is doubling every 14 months, thus keeping pace with infection rates among homosexuals and intravenous drug users. The report said, "The number of increases in the heterosexual cases is proportional to the increases in other risk groups."

"Heterosexual spread (of AIDS) in the U.S. has become a reality," said Dr. King Holmes, a venereologist at the Seattle Harbor View Medical Center. "It appears that AIDS has spread through the general population where it was initially dismissed as 'AIDS hysteria.' "

University of California epidemiologist Nancy Padian gave a startling and thoroughly sobering report. She said, "Condom use and number of lifetime sexual partners and sexually-transmitted diseases have no apparent effect on HIV transmission risk." This is contradictory to the Masters and Johnson report and even more ominous.

About one third of the estimated 1.5 million Americans infected with AIDS are heterosexuals.[3] Several speakers at the Stockholm conference on AIDS presented more evidence that the AIDS virus is continuing to spread into heterosexual populations.

Dr. H. Hunter Handsfield, director of the sexually transmitted disease control program for the Seattle-King County Department of Public Health, said during a discussion session at the Stockholm meeting that he had not expected heterosexual-transmission to become as serious a problem as it now appears to be. He said, "My mind is being changed in bits and pieces... I'm very impressed by some of the data in the last few days and very nervous about it." One wonders if Dr. Windom and Dr. Koop are not also getting nervous.

---

3   Internal Medicine News, July, 15-31, 1987.

Dr. Windom's flat statement that AIDS is not entering the heterosexual community sounds strange indeed in light of the report from the highly respected *New England Journal of Medicine (NEJM)* which said, "...Numerous studies in Africa, Haiti and the United States have made it clear that heterosexual-transmission is probably the leading route of HIV infection worldwide *and is increasingly important in the United States.*"

The *NEJM* concluded, "...The proportion of AIDS cases in this country that are attributable to heterosexual transmission is increasing more rapidly than the proportion of cases in any other category of risk."

A Johns Hopkins University survey in Baltimore Maryland, revealed that half the women who tested positive for AIDS and a third of the men were not homosexuals, did *not* use drugs and were *not* promiscuous. That doesn't help the Surgeon General's fairy tale: "You can't catch AIDS through casual contact."

It is possible that even the government propaganda concerning intravenous drug use may be a red herring. If the intravenous route is the easiest way to catch AIDS, why does it take as long as five to seven years for some recipients of contaminated blood to come down with AIDS? Is it not possible that in the interim from the time of transfusion until contracting AIDS, they got it from some other source?

The city of Los Angeles has as many intravenous drug addicts as the city of New York, but they have a very low rate of infection with AIDS.4 Statistics reported at the Third Annual International AIDS Conference revealed that 61 percent of New York drug abusers test positive for AIDS, but only 15 percent test positive in southern California and zero percent are positive in Tampa, Florida, and San Antonio, Texas.

---

4   Los Angeles Times, 11/21/87.

Irene Raymond contracted AIDS from a blood transfusion she received seven years ago. Before she realized her diagnosis she had given AIDS to her husband, her six-year-old daughter Claire, their three-year-old daughter Rachel and their 20-months-old daughter Danielle. Only the Raymond's son, Stuart, has thus far escaped this tragedy.5 Yet we are told that family members of AIDS patients are perfectly safe.

Surgeon General Koop's favorite criticism of people with whom he disagrees is to call them "irresponsible." I have received this criticism from him as have Doctors Masters and Johnson. Masters and Johnson said in the conclusion to their book: "AIDS is breaking out. The AIDS virus is now running rampant in the heterosexual community. Unless something is done to contain this global epidemic, we face a mounting death toll in the years ahead that will be the most formidable the world has ever seen."

Adding credence to the Masters and Johnson report is the finding at the Lake County, Indiana, jail. Dr. Alphonso Holliday, the jail medical director, said that he had been ready to stop testing his inmates for the AIDS virus in 1986. They found "only one case in 663 tested."

"We thought it was just a whole lot of noise," he said. However, they then found that the AIDS-infection rate at the Crown Point jail was skyrocketing. *One in every 67 inmates tested positive for the virus.* Then the situation became even worse, and from July through September, 1988, *one of every 40* inmates tested positive for the AIDS virus.

"The statistics indicate what's in the community. It's not an epidemic in the jail. *You've got an epidemic in the community,*" Dr. Holliday remarked.

---

5 The People (London), 8/21/88.

Dr. Robert Gallo has reported, "The risk of hetero-sexual-transmission cannot yet be assessed, and the future rates of infection of the heterosexual population for most parts of the world cannot be predicted."[6]

Many experts disagree with Doctors Koop and Windom. Doctors Victor D. Gruttola and Kenneth H. Mayer of the Harvard School of Medicine reported in the *Reviews of Infectious Diseases:* "The fact that the proportion of cases resulting from heterosexual contact is small and will probably remain so for the next several years does not appear to preclude the subsequent development of a major epidemic among heterosexuals."[7]

Dr. Robert R. Redfield of the Walter Reed Army Institute of Research reported, "In light of our current understanding of the prolonged asymptomatic period of infection, focusing on AIDS cases allows accurate estimation only of the historic epidemiology of viral transmission five to ten years ago .... The actual magnitude of the problem today can only be determined by focusing on the extent of (AIDS) infection, not AIDS."[8]

Perhaps even more impressive in giving the lie to government propaganda about heterosexual AIDS is the report on AIDS in pregnant women in New York City. A study in 1987 found that the highest rates of AIDS were among pregnant women. There is little argument, even among the most radical groups, that if a woman is pregnant it's ipso facto evidence that she's probably heterosexual. The study reported in *Annals of Internal Medicine* reveals some very bizarre findings. The older the woman the more likely she was to be infected with the AIDS virus. None of the women under 24 years of age were infected, yet 7.1 percent of women over the age of 31 were infected with AIDS.

6 Gallo and Wong-Staal, *Nature*, 10/3/85.
7 *Reviews of Infectious Diseases,* January-February, 1988.
8 *Mt. Sinai Journal of Medicine,* December 1986.

"These women were characterized by heterosexual activity and fertility," the report noted, "in contrast to intravenous drug use or prostitution, and may more closely reflect the HIV sero-prevalence in a heterogeneous population of sexually active women in New York City..." This survey suggests high existing levels of HIV infection of women in their middle and late twenties. (The infection rate went from zero in women under 24 to 7.7 percent in women from 26 to 30 years of age, and then to 7.1 percent in women over 31.)[9]

In the conclusion to their book, Masters and Johnson also said: "The somewhat chilling conclusion we have reached is this: the AIDS VH us has certainly established a beachhead in the ranks of heterosexuals, and because heterosexuals who have large numbers of sex partners are most likely to be infected, the odds are that the rate of spread among heterosexuals will now begin to escalate at a frightening pace."

Dr. William A. Haseltine of the Harvard School of Public Health reinforces the opinions of Masters and Johnson: "Many experts fear that, if the AIDS virus has gained a 'beachhead' in the heterosexual population of the   United States, the experience in Africa could be repeated here. We don't understand the conditions for heterosexual spread in Africa enough to predict that it cann'ot happen in our major urban centers as well .... The potential is there, and the burden of proof should be placed on those who claimed it will not spread. *It is foolhardy to think that what happened in Africa could not happen here.*"[10] (Emphasis added.)

The statistics clearly point to the veracity and credence of Dr. Haseltine's report. Heterosexual cases of AIDS are now rapidly increasing and at a rate much

9   *Annals of Internal Medicine,* October 1987.
10 *Washington Post,* 3/15/88.

faster than in the homosexual community. According to the Centers for Disease Control, in 1986 heterosexual contact cases grew by 136 percent as compared to 82 percent among homosexuals.

It's highly significant that there is a skyrocketing increase in sexually-transmitted diseases such as syphilis, gonorrhea, human papilloma virus, herpes, etc. As these sexual diseases *have a much shorter incubation period than AIDS*, this would indicate that in five to ten years many, if not most, of these infected people will come down with AIDS ("Herpes now—AIDS later"). The Washington School of Medicine reports that the risk of spreading AIDS is eight times as high if the carrier suffers from some type of genital sore such as herpes or syphilitic chancre.

Dr. Thomas C. Quinn said at the Inter-Science Conference on Anti-Microbial Agents and Chemotherapy, that one-third of the men and nearly one-half of the women in his practice became infected through heterosexual contact. He said, "These are very big numbers... that's one in 20 people that's coming through the door, and these people are having sex with everyone else."

Although Dr. Quinn said he was surprised to find such high rates among heterosexuals, and 48 percent of the women denied any risk factor, and 40 percent of the men denied the same, he repeated the old mantra of the government propagandists that "HIV does not appear to be spreading to heterosexuals who do not have a known risk factor"![11]

The most impressive corroboration of the Masters and Johnson report thus far is the study done by the highly respected Hudson Institute. This report, because it very strongly supports Masters and Johnson, will undoubtedly be stone-walled by the government and the news media.

---

11 *Internal Medicine News*, December 1-14,1987.

173

Dr. George A. Keyworth, director of research at the Hudson Institute, characterized the report as a "sober warning to the AIDS skeptics. Even though no one knows for certain how many people in the United States are infected, this report pointedly suggests that we may be gravely underestimating the extent of the epidemic, especially among heterosexuals. The disease may be spreading much faster than has been generally believed.

"If there is a large pool of infected people," Keyworth continued, "then there are important new implications for national health policy—not only in terms of the strain on medical treatment resources, but also in terms of the potential spread of the disease in coming years."

The Hudson Institute report pointed out that *"the lack of a sophisticated understanding of the spread of the HIV infection might well be the most dangerous gap in our knowledge about AIDS."*

The Institute report quoted Dr. William Haseltine of the Boston Dana-Farber Institute:

"We do not have an accurate view of the number of infected people in the United States, or indeed anywhere in the world, because no representative measurement of our population has been done. The tools for the determination of the infection of the population have been available for three years. It is a major failure of government's response to the epidemic that a cross sectional survey of the population for HIV-I infection is not completed... At present, we are 'flying blind' with respect to this fundamental aspect of the epidemic."

The Hudson Institute report makes some simple but very obvious points about the spread of AIDS which everyone is choosing to ignore. They point out that the only reliable indicator of the true size of the AIDS epidemic is not the number of AIDS cases, but rather the *number of people infected with the virus*—both those who display the symptoms of AIDS as well as those who show no signs of the disease.

The most popular method at present of determining the severity of the epidemic is to take a particular group, say homosexuals of San Francisco, determine the number of active cases, divide it by the total population in that area, which gives you a true percentage figure. If you take that percentage and multiply it by the total number of cases in the United States you come up with a total number of presumed cases among that group in the United States. This method is very crude and actually has very little meaning. As the Hudson Institute report points out, "The major problem with this type of estimation is that it assumes that the number of infected persons bears a constant relationship, both over time and geographically, to the number of AIDS cases. There is no theoretical or empirical reason for this to be so. In fact, the opposite is more likely to be true ...."

The Hudson Institute quotes Jeffrey Harris of MIT: *"Actually, one hundred million people can be infected right now and it could be complete) compatible with the current data on the epidemic, because none of them would have gotten AIDS yet."*

"We simply do not know," the Institute says, "within any reasonably close approximation, how many people are infected with HIV... and yet, despite this critical lack of information, the conventional wisdom has made its way firmly into the popular understanding... and has become an unjustifiable, and perhaps dangerously wrong, basis for national debate and policy-making in the battle against AIDS."

Studies have shown, the report says, that fully nine percent of people with no known exposure to HIV infection and testing negative on the conventional probe are nonetheless found to be harboring the virus. They con-

175

clude, "...This result makes the serial prevalence surveys conducted to date almost useless ...."

Although the Hudson Institute report is based primarily on good statistical analysis, they make some extremely cogent social comments concerning AIDS among the heterosexual population.

"...Because of the high incidence of divorce and breakdowns of non-marital but otherwise monogamous relationships, heterosexuals move frequently into and out of the non-monogamous sexually-active pool of persons, even if, for a time, they are theoretically insulated from exposure to the virus through celibacy or monogamy.

"There also are a great number of avenues for heterosexuals to become infected. *Many gay or bi-sexual men have sex regular} with heterosexual women as well as with men....*

"...Most of the people who currently have AIDS and who are heterosexual have been infected for about ten years and have been transmitting the virus to their partners throughout this period."

In stark contrast to the supposed two percent of American heterosexuals who are reported to have the AIDS virus, among the adjusted total of these cases diagnosed through the end of 1987, *"nearly one-third were heterosexuals."*

Surgeon General Koop admitted that he had not read the Masters and Johnson book. Has he read the Hudson Institute report? Has Dr. Robert E. Windom, Dr. Koop's assistant, who states categorically that AIDS is not spreading into the heterosexual community, read *either* of these reports?

One hesitates to call anyone a liar. But what can be said of two men in such exalted positions in Public Health making such statements in the face of the evidence that we have presented? Is our government being held captive by certain powerful minority groups that make it politically impossible for these men to *tell* the truth? Would it not be the honorable thing for them to resign and speak out before it is too late' Shouldn't they do this, if for no other reason, than just for the good of their own families?

Chapter 9
A Vaccination for AIDS

It is ironic that the great AIDS plague was brought upon man through vaccination—a smallpox vaccination campaign in Africa, Brazil and Haiti, and by the use of the Hepatitis-B vaccine on homosexuals in the United States (See Chapter 4.) Now we are to expect the very people who created this international holocaust to save us with *another* vaccination.

Some important questions need answering:

(1) Can we expect these scientists, with their abysmal track record, to help us?

(2) Will it be possible to make a vaccine against the AIDS virus?

(3) Do vaccinations really work?

The first question is difficult to answer. It would seem, at first glance, that the microbiologists are the ones to whom we should turn. But they are taking us ever deeper into a complicated and disastrous course in which a Pandora's box has been opened, thus releasing bacteria and viruses that are more dangerous than anything ever conceived by nature. The microbiologists are committed to Louis Pasteur, i.e. vaccination, and they cannot shake off the shackles of tradition and look at more promising avenues such as electro-magnetic medicine.

The quest for fame and fortune, although not bad or necessarily counter-productive per se, has goaded scientists toward pursuing great reputations and even greater riches by going down the traditional lines of research. Dr. William Haseltine, for instance, holds shares in Cambridge BioScience worth about $4.7 million. Haseltine, a born promoter and entrepreneur, set up Cambridge Bio-

Science and invited his colleague, Myron Essex of Harvard) to become an exclusive consultant to Haseltine's new money machine.

Haseltine once said, "Ask my friends. I predicted (AIDS) 10 or 15 years ago." With the sinister origins of the AIDS virus, I am not sure that I would want to brag about that. Did Haseltine merely read the right issue of the Bulletin of the World Health Organization[1] in which the engineering of the AIDS virus was proposed? Did he know scientists in the World Health Organization who were working on developing the AIDS virus? Did Haseltine take part in these experiments?

Remarking on Dr. Haseltine's prescience, a magazine stated: "The assertion of a new virus was an extraordinarily prescient piece of science, the importance of which cannot be over-estimated."[2] Was it prescience or did Haseltine know something the rest of us did not?

Haseltine's partner "Max" Essex became famous by coming to some incorrect conclusions. Essex thought that the AIDS virus was a retrovirus akin to certain leukemia viruses. He was correct about AIDS being a retrovirus, but he was wrong on all the rest. But being half right secured him the undisputed mantle of the prophet of AIDS.

Essex, like another of his colleagues, Robert Gallo, is somewhat of a scientific gadfly. As a magazine described him, "His faith appears to be not so much in the rigors of science as in himself, and while it has led to great triumphs ... it is also the result of his failures."[3] Essex and his friend Gallo clung to the idea that AIDS was a leukemia-causing virus even after the discovery of the HIV virus by the French. Essex, Gallo and

---

1 Allison, et. al., *Bull*. WHO 1972,47:257-63 and Amos, et.al.; Fed. Proc. 1972,31:1087.
2 *New England Monthly*, June, 1988.
3 Ibid.

Haseltine began to take on the aura of car salesmen pushing their own line of products, in this case the HTLV virus line. Gallo, Haseltine and Essex are now in positions of tremendous power, being able to dictate where the grant and research money goes, who gets published and who doesn't.

Haseltine, with 350 thousand shares of stock in his company, is clearly in conflict of interest when he serves on various editorial boards (five scientific journals) and many scientific committees–nine at the last count. Incidentally, three of these committees favor money for AIDS research.

All three of these men are scientific hustlers, but there is no question that Haseltine is the lead huskey.

"We see a wave of devastating disease approaching ...." The prognosis—careful measured, authoritative—filled the crowded Senate hearing room, as it was meant to, as a clarion call. "The magnitude and nature of the problem is crystal clear." Bill Haseltine had not been a national figure before and was hardly known outside a relatively small community of microbiologists who would normally be the only ones to care about or understand what he had to say. But his speech to the Senate Appropriations Sub-Committee in September of 1985 urging dramatically increased federal support in the fight against AIDS was as much a breakthrough as Essex's discovery of GP120, the "docking protein" of the AIDS virus.

Haseltine, as it turned out, had a gift for talking about AIDS in a manner both relentlessly dire and upbeat. He could explain the disease in its most depressing details, yet convey such competence about bio-medicine's ability to fight it that he left one feeling exhilarated, even hopeful. He was the ideal spokesman. The media, ever eager for a simple take-home message in the mountains of data and counter-data they were being asked to comprehend, sought him out. Presidential campaign staffs asked his advice. Lay funding agencies coveted his counsel. "That Bill Haseltine," a cab driver at Logan Airport would announce–unsolicited–to another scientist, "That's the guy I listen to."[4]

The position of power that these three men hold has created a great deal of resentment and animosity among the scientific community. Dr. Michael Lange, assistant head of infectious diseases, St. Luke's Hospital, said, "We've lost three years in AIDS drug development... because of the Gallo/Essex/Haseltine axis boycotting other ideas."

This triumvirate of egotistical and greedy doctors has made a mockery of the idea of common cause in science. Scientists cannot work alone on an island. There must be a spirit of cooperation with everyone's talent and discoveries being used to come to the ultimate objective of solving a scientific problem. The trio have successfully driven some promising young researchers from the field, brooking no possible threat to their preeminence and control of AIDS research. Priority obsessed, they have refused to share what they know and have thrown roadblocks in the way of those who might disagree with them.

One scientist found that he was denied reagents from a commercial laboratory. He &covered that the only way to get along was to "make a deal" as you would if you were bargaining for camels.

Dr. David Baltimore, Nobel prize winner and apparently not part of this money-making machine, said, "I believe we are in a national emergency, and the biomedical community will be judged in the future by how we respond."

One bitter scientist said, "Maybe we should give each of the researchers on AIDS a million dollars—and then demand: 'now stop acting like a greedy bugger and get on with the job.' "

---

4 *New England Monthly*, June, 1988.

Will companies like Cambridge BioScience, as with the American Cancer Society, develop such a vested interest searching for a cure for AIDS that a cure will never be found?

The "war against AIDS" has become so commercial that even parts of the AIDS virus are now being patented. Myron Essex, a big stockholder in Cambridge BioScience Corporation, discovered the now-patented protein, GP120, from the AIDS virus and has it tucked away snugly in his Worchester, Massachusetts, operation.

Harvard administrators, correctly, were concerned about a potential conflict of interest between Essex, BioScience and Harvard. But Essex says he "has not paid much attention to the financial potential of his research." It is hard to imagine that one would not notice two million dollars worth of stock, especially when you are in a position to control the destiny of that company through your association with Harvard University.

Hiram Caton of the Division of Humanities at Griffith University, Brisbane, Australia, has made some serious and timely charges against the appalling AIDS research industry that has developed, especially in the United States.

"Despite the huge uncertainties of the nature of the disease," he said, "its transmission and effects and about the financial, legal and moral dilemmas surrounding society's response, scientists and health authorities present a united voice for a single policy option, which they vigorously defend as the only rational and humane policy." The "single policy option," to which Hiram Caton is referring, is a vaccine.

David Baltimore, who has piously announced that microbiologists will be judged concerning how they handle the AIDS epidemic, is not entirely free of mean-spirited control over competitors. In 1986 the U.S. National Academy of Sciences presented a report called "Confronting

AIDS." At a press conference at which the report was re-leased, the co-chairman David Baltimore declared: "Any alternative to the report's preferred preventive policy was inconceivable."

As Dr. Caton said, "In functional terms, Baltimore's statement is a warning to scientists who might examine the report in a critical spirit. In doing so they incur the displeasure of the establishment that controls research funding prestige. Very few American scientists have strayed from the fold.

"Self-deception and truth management," Caton ar-gued, "are endemic among scientists as in other works of life. Eminent scientists of undoubted integrity are liable to confect transparently bogus and biased reading of evi-dence."[5]

A prime example of the sleazy and clearly dishonest activities in Cambridge BioScience is the marketing of their AIDS virus test.

The company has now acknowledged at a conference in Stockholm in the summer of 1988[6] that it blocked an outside group from publishing unfavorable data about its experimental diagnostic test for AIDS.

A test program was sponsored by the Program for Corporate Technology and Health, acronym PATH, a nonprofit Seattle-based group that researches medical technology. The study compared results among some four thousand patients with five different new tests for diagnosing AIDS. The Cambridge BioScience tests per-formed worse than the other tests, some of which de-tected antibodies to the AIDS virus in 98 percent or more of the patients who had them.[7]

---

5 *New Scientist*, 26 May 1988.
6 *Wall Street Journal*, 6/21/B8.
7 *Daily News*, 11/21188.

Although the Cambridge BioScience test proved to be mediocre at best, it is being marketed in several European and African countries and is now approved in the United States. Altruism and true science obviously go out the window when you are dealing with an $18 million a year market (and rising).[8]

So the question about finding help from these virologists must be answered with a very tentative "maybe." To our second question about the feasibility of a vaccine, we need to look at the work of veterinarians who have been attempting to find a vaccine against retroviruses for about 50 years. AIDS, a recombinant retrovirus from animals, is the first of these retroviruses ever to infect man.

Although they have been working on the problem since retroviruses were first identified in animals, *vets have never been successful in developing a successful vaccine against any form of retrovirus, not one.* When visna virus decimated the sheep population of Iceland, an attempt was made to vaccinate the healthy animals remaining. It was a complete failure, and every sheep on the island had to be slaughtered.

What this means is that all the testing of animals for an AIDS-like vaccine has been done before—and failed.

The story of vaccines and vaccination in relation to AIDS would not be complete without some mention of the swine flu immunization fiasco of 1977-78.

Although most Americans have forgotten or are not aware of the terrible devastation caused by the swine flu epidemic of 1918-19, most public health officials are very attuned to that epidemic because it killed 500,000 Americans. Twenty million people died worldwide. It was the worst medical disaster in the history of modern medicine. Thoughts of the return of this terrible plague are never far from the minds of public health experts.

---

8 Ibid.

So when swine flu, or what was thought to be swine flu, broke out in a small epidemic at Fort Dix, New Jersey, public health officials jumped to a lot of unwarranted conclusions. There was set in motion the greatest public health fiasco in the history of the United States.

Although the virus which caused the 1918-19 pandemic was never identified with certainty, public health officials at the Centers For Disease Control became convinced, without any further evidence, that we were facing the return of the great flu plague for the flu season of 1977-78. Although no new "swine flu" cases were discovered at Fort Dix after the initial outbreak, or anywhere else in the United States for that matter–or even in the world–the Centers For Disease Control and its brash and extremely aggressive head, Dr. David Sencer, began a headlong rush into disaster.

Most experts said that a swine flu epidemic of the proportions of the 1918-19 epidemic was highly unlikely and, considering that immunization attempts against the flu epidemics of 1957 and 1968 had been completely unsuccessful, it was felt that this would be a very expensive, and possibly dangerous fool's errand by the CDC.

Although the CDC and Sencer were hell-bent for immunization of the entire population against swine flu, an unprecedented public health measure, there were some cool heads warning against such an ambitious project. Dr. E. Russell Alexander, Professor of Public Health at the University of Washington, said: "Our general view is that you should be conservative about putting foreign material into the human body. That's always true... especially when you are talking about two hundred million bodies. The need should be estimated conservatively. If you don't need to give it, don't."[9]

---

9 Nestadt and Fineberg, *The Swine Flu Affair*, p. 12.

185

But CDC officials were assuring everyone, in Dr. Walter Dowdle's words, that the vaccine was perfectly safe – just like water."

Sencer, a clever politician, assembled his staff of "experts" to sandbag President Gerald Ford into approving the program and putting his stamp of approval on it. Included in this group were both Doctors Jonas Salk and Albert Sabin, the developers of the two polio vaccines. Notably absent from the committee was Dr. E. Russell Alexander, whom we quoted above as being opposed to the vaccination.

Doctors Salk and Sabin both enthusiastically supported vaccination, even though no one would even attempt to assess the actual danger of an epidemic. Not one of the members of the panel spoke up against the massive immunization program or expressed any doubts whatsoever. The "Sencership" was complete.

The President was ambushed into making his decision based on the recommendations of this stacked panel. As one of the participants on the panel said after the fact, "I regretted not having spoken up and said, 'Mr. President, this may not be proper for me to say, but I believe we should not go ahead with immunization until we are sure this is a real threat.' " Even Sencer himself admitted that it was merely a rubber stamp conference. It was so cut and dried that while the scientists were consulting with the President, government press officials were passing out the swine flu "fact sheets" bearing the message that the President would deliver at the conclusion of the meeting. At 4:50 PM Ford appeared at the White House press room, flanked by Doctors Sabin and Salk, and announced that the mass immunization would take place.

Although the President was literally tricked into recommending this program, as a politician he naturally would appreciate the benefits that would accrue from taking the lead in protecting the public from this great scourge. His pleasure was short-lived.

The evening news erupted with opinions from that part of the scientific community that had not been heard at this meeting. Walter Cronkite reported, "Some doctors and public health officials ... believe that such a massive program is premature and unwise, that there is not enough proof of the need for it ... but because President Ford and others are endorsing the program, those who oppose it privately are afraid to say so in public."

The program was called "crazy," "rotten to the core," "unwarranted" and "politically-inspired."

The vaccine is made from the yolks of eggs, and a certain number of people could be expected to have violent allergic reactions to the chicken product. This would turn out to be the least of their problems. The American Medical Association, always in the forefront of any type of immunization drive, strongly supported the program but would soon, like the Public Health establishment, have a lot of egg on its face.

Although Dr. Cooper of the CDC was assuring everyone that the vaccine would be 90 percent effective and have little or no side effects, wiser heads knew there was still considerable controversy about the effectiveness of any influenza vaccine, including the swine flu. In fact, the CDC itself had done a study in 1968-69 which proved that, "optimally constituted influenza vaccines at standard dosage levels have little, if any, effectiveness ...." This was certainly confirmed at Fort Dix, where there was an epidemic of Victoria flu as well as the so-called swine flu and, although vaccinated, many of the recruits came down with the victoria flu anyway.

Dr. Martin Goldfield, a New Jersey epidemiologist, came out adamantly against the program. He said, "When we talk emotionally about gambling with lives, we must also remember that we are gambling with health

187

and welfare if we throw around two hundred million doses of the vaccine.

...There are as many dangers in going ahead with immunizing the population as there are in withholding."

The Office of Management and Budget (OMB), which had been against the massive vaccination campaign from the beginning, suggested that the White House and the CDC re-think their program. "The main reason for a possible change in approach, is that there have not been any further cases of swine flu *anywhere* in the world since the 12 Fort Dix cases in February .... There is no available evidence to demonstrate that the 1976 version of swine flu is any more virulent than any other current strains of flu."

In spite of this finding of no flu anywhere, and the emphasis on "anywhere" was in the original report from the OMB, and the fact that the southern hemisphere which was right in the middle of the flu season and experiencing practically no flu, the political juggernaut was on its way and the President was politically committed.

Matters got rapidly worse. Incredibly, the planners forgot to allow in the trials for a two-dose regimen for children, those considered most vulnerable to the virus and those most likely to spread the infection. One field worker later admitted, "We just didn't think of it." (!)

Adding to the chaos, the highly respected Parke-Davis Pharmaceutical Company, which was producing a great percentage of the vaccine for the program, had somehow *used the wrong virus.* Millions of doses of this inappropriate vaccine had to be discarded, which set the program back another six weeks.

No one seemed to notice (or wanted to notice) that the virus yield was only one vaccine dose per egg, which would indicate that their Fort Dix swine flu was a non-virulent form which was very unlikely to cause a pandemic. It was also noted, but quietly ignored, that the vaccine worked very poorly in children, those who would be in most need of the vaccine if, in fact, an effective vaccine was ever manufactured.

Because of the failure to provide proper testing in the young and the simple observation that the vaccine didn't work in them anyway, children were excluded from the program without the American people being told. It was felt by officials, and rightly so, an admission that children were not being included in the program could be considered gross malfeasance and a demonstration of total incompetence.

By June of 1976 it was becoming clearly apparent, due to the lack of any epidemic in the southern hemisphere, that there would not be anything even approaching a flu epidemic. Dr. Sabin backed out, reversed himself and urged that the program be discontinued.

By late July it was being admitted by a high official in the Centers For Disease Control that there was probably no need for the vaccination program. The assistant director of the CDC said, "We have no reason to raise the spectre of 1918 in connection with the Fort Dix incident."

Now everyone was beginning to back off except, of course, the Centers For Disease Control. Something very strange happened which seems to illustrate how illogical and dangerous human beings can be when making decisions on the basis of mass emotion—including the Congress of the United States.

Legionnaire's Disease burst upon the scene in Philadelphia and the President used this outbreak to convince Congress to put their stamp of approval on the swine flu vaccination program. The President told Congress that although the tragic deaths in Philadelphia were not caused by the swine flu, he said, "But let us remember one thing: they could have been!" With this peculiar logic in hand Congress overwhelmingly passed the swine flu immunization program.

189

Adding to this incredible fiasco, it was discovered that all of the vaccines being produced lacked a key component, a surface protein, that contributes greatly to the vaccine's effectiveness. This meant that the vaccine was, even to those who believed in vaccines, probably useless. But the program went relentlessly forward to disaster.

Contributing to this mess, the Centers For Disease Control stated falsely in forms given out with the vaccine that it "can be taken safely during pregnancy." It had not even been tested on pregnant women. It was also unclear to the vaccinees that the "registration form" the CDC was handing out was actually an "informed consent," giving the government permission to administer the vaccine. The CDC omitted to inform people that the epidemic was far from certain or that the vaccine was probably going to be totally ineffective due to leaving out the surface protein. Risks were minimized and likely benefits were subtly exaggerated. This type of conduct by the Centers For Disease Control is the sort of thing that would cause a private practitioner to lose his license for quackery.

Even more important, the forms warning of certain possible side effects completely omitted the possibility of any neurological complications, even though the four manufacturers of the vaccine had been careful to include this information. The association between all flu vaccines and neurologic illness was well-known and established.

When three elderly people dropped dead shortly after receiving the swine flu shots in Pittsburgh, Pennsylvania, the program was temporarily closed down, and nine states quickly followed suit. This prompted the New York Times to editorialize that the President should "order a halt in the vaccination program until there had been a second hard look at the cost and benefits of what is being done to forestall the disease that isn't there."

The panic subsided when President Ford and his family got their flu shots on national television, and the mass immunization program proceeded. However, federal officials suggested that the advertising council handling the publicity for the immunization program leave off the tag line that had been planned "Swine flu shot. Get it Before It Gets You."

Many Americans did indeed think that the swine flu vaccination would "get them" and in some states the participation was as low as 12 percent. Fortunately for the American people they remained skeptical about the need, the efficacy and the safety of the vaccine.

The manufacture of the wrong virus by Parke-Davis, the leaving out of important proteins, the misrepresentation to the public about safety in pregnancy, the lack of proper testing for children, the covering up on warning labels of the possibility of side effects, especially neurological diseases, and the lack of any real evidence of the approach of any kind of epidemic, were all bad enough, but then came the really bad news—an epidemic of paralysis, called Guillain-Barrpé syndrome, caused by the vaccine. After a thousand cases of this paralysis had been reported, the CDC had reluctantly to admit that they were indeed related to the vaccine. Dr. Cooper of the CDC, emphasizing that this was only a temporary cessation, announced a suspension of the swine flu program: "...in the interest of the safety of the public... of credibility and... of the practice of good medicine," the program was discontinued—never to be seen again.

The government's public health image has never recovered and is not likely to in the near future. The present urging by the CDC of elderly people to take the current fad "flu shots" will probably fall on very wary and suspicious ears.

It chilling to think that this organization, the Centers For Disease Control, are supposed to be one of the major governmental organizations protecting us from the ravages of AIDS. As Diana B. Dutton says in her book, **Worse Than the Disease—Pitfalls of Medical Progress,** "Their failure highlights the danger of relying; too heavily on the views of technical experts, whose unswerving confidence in the safety and efficacy of medical intervention (even in the name of prevention) seems to blind them to impending problems and of insulating national health policy from public scrutiny."

This vaccine disaster should be kept in mind by Americans who are being told that you can't catch AIDS through casual contact; you can't catch it from mosquitoes; and that you simply will not catch AIDS period, unless you are engaging in some unusual, socially unacceptable behavior.

One CDC official suggested, after the debacle was complete, "The flu program should be considered the 'Viet Nam of the Public Health Service' and that at some point victory should be claimed and we should pull out."[10] In other words, more "Sencership."

Since the influenza epidemic following World War I, microbiologists have been attempting to perfect an influenza vaccine that really works. They have failed on every try, although Americans are still urged to take their annual flu shots in spite of the swine flu vaccine disaster. They are of no value because the flu virus that comes around the second year will be entirely different from the one from the previous year. So even if the principle of vaccination is valid, and many have their doubts, it is not feasible to make a vaccine to hit a moving target.

The primary benefactor of today's needle brigade is our elderly citizens. There is a massive propaganda campaign underway to convince people over 65 that they need to take a "flu shot" to avoid serious disease, hospi-

---

10 Bernstein, *The Swine Flu Immunization Program*, a quote of Jay Davenport: "Flu Staff Meeting," 11/10/76.

talization and even death. F. L. Ruben of the University of Pittsburgh's Medical School, said, "We must draw a ring of immunity around our senior citizens."

In spite of this bold and idealistic proclamation, Dr. William Schaffner, chief of infectious diseases at Vanderbilt University School of Medicine said, "We're always looking into a cloudy crystal ball...."

A five-year study at a British boarding school revealed that influenza was no more prevalent among students who never got a shot than it was among those who were vaccinated every year. Many children got sick throughout the five years in spite of receiving annual flu shots.

With the elderly, the odds are as high as 50 percent that they will get influenza in spite of the shot. Nancy Arden, an epidemiologist for the Centers for Disease Control, has admitted that "the U.S. policy is not to try to decrease the incidence of disease, which is practically impossible, but to prevent severe complications and deaths." These are interesting admissions, but there are far more serious questions.

In view of the fact that polio vaccine, given to millions of children and young adults in the 1960s, was contaminated with a monkey virus which causes cancer,11 what assurance do we have that influenza vaccines do not contain a similar cancer-causing virus?

What animal tissue was used to grow the new influenza vaccine? Have the vaccines been carefully tested to rule out a cancer-causing virus from the animal tissue used? Have the animals used, presumably monkeys, to test the safety of the vaccines lived out their normal life span? If so, how many of these animals came down with some form of cancer?

---

11 *New England Journal of Medicine*, 1972, 286,:385.

Dr. John Seale of London has observed that the simian virus-40 from African monkeys, when contracted by Asiatic monkeys, whether accidentally or by injection, they come down with virulent, rapidly fatal cancer. The virus has little effect on its original host, the green monkey. Are we possibly, with the flu vaccine program, inoculating millions of Americans with a similar animal virus that, although innocuous to its host, will cause virulent cancer in humans? Will serial passaging of this virus in humans through the years produce a more rapidly fatal type of cancer, as has been known to happen in other vaccine experiments?

If monkey virus-contaminated polio vaccine was the fiasco of the 60s, the fiasco of the 70s was the rubella (German measles) vaccination program. Superimposed over these vaccination follies is the *continuing fiasco* of influenza immunization.

The German measles vaccine has an interesting history in that four different animal types of cells have been used in its investigation and manufacture: monkey kidney, rabbit kidney, dog kidney and duck embryo. All these animals, especially monkey, rabbit and duck, can harbor highly virulent forms of cancer. The myxoma virus of rabbits is as fatal as AIDS and, if modified for human consumption through serial passage, could be as devastating as an AIDS infection, except that death would probably come quicker.

The original inventors of the rubella vaccine, Doctors Meyer and Parkman, passaged the virus 74 times through some animal tissue culture, and then pronounced that they had an effective vaccine against rubella.

Keeping in mind the tragedy of the polio monkey-contaminated vaccine, is it possible that after 73 transfers there might be other viruses going along for the ride? As many of these viral contaminants which cause cancer have an incubation period of up to 40 years, it will be well into the twenty-first century before we know whether these children will come down with cancer when in young or middle adulthood.

Doctors Meyer and Parkman announced that their monkeys, when inoculated, had produced antibodies to German measles and had not transmitted the disease. After 73 passages, the virus has been completely transformed from a human virus to a monkey virus. Therefore it *should* now infect monkeys. This is the reverse of the manufacture of the AIDS virus where animal viruses, through passage, were converted to a human virus. Because of the species barrier which prevents animal viruses generally from infecting humans, the newly created monkey recombinant theoretical) shouldn't cause disease in humans But our experience with Simian Virus-40 and polio vaccine makes one uneasy.

Again the question must be asked, concerning these experimental animals, were the monkeys sacrificed or left to live out their normal life span? If they lived their normal life span, how many of them developed cancer? Did they develop any other debilitating diseases such as an MS type disease or arthritis? Did they die prematurely? As sheets of duck cells were used to manufacture the rubella vaccine, was the vaccine tested carefully for viral contaminants from ducks?

In their first testing of their vaccine, Meyer and Parkman went to an Arkansas School for the Mentally Retarded in Conway, Arkansas. Although they claim that this initial study was a great success, it would be interesting to know what has happened to those children in the past 20 years. Has there been a follow-up? What is the incidence of cancer or other degenerative diseases among these children? How many premature deaths were there? Until these questions are answered the vaccine certainly cannot be proclaimed as safe. Even 20 years may not be long enough because of the 40-year incubation of some lethal viruses.

Jean Carper, in her article, "The Race Against Rubella," **World Book Encyclopedia**, 1970, said that after the vaccine was "perfected" healthy children were "challenged" to see if, after an inoculation, they would contract German measles. Vaccinated subjects were given inhalations of the wild virus. She reports that the children did not get rubella. However, she does not indicate that any control was done where children who had not received the vaccine were also challenged. Did unvaccinated children get rubella?

Acute rheumatoid-type arthritis is a quite common complication of German measles infection. It would be interesting to know, after a 20 year follow-up, how many of these children developed chronic rheumatoid arthritis or other arthritic diseases.

Some researchers are now taking a serious look at the rubella-German measles vaccine and wondering out loud if it might not be responsible for the chronic fatigue syndrome which is now devastating millions of young Americans. The condition is also called, probably mistakenly, the Epstein-Barr syndrome.

The rubella vaccine was received with great fanfare by public health officials when introduced. The vaccine, because it is a live virus, is dangerous and fraught with unpredictable results. We seem to have learned nothing from the swine flu disaster.

The problem, as Allen Alan of Algorithms, Inc., sees it, is that the virus lives in vaccinated children for years and "can be transmitted easily to others through a touch, a cough or a kiss."[12] The originators of the vaccine assured us their experiments had proven that vaccinated children would not transmit the virus to others.[13] Twenty years of experience have proven this not to be true.

---

12 *UPI*, 12/30)87
13 **World Book Encyclopedia,** 1970.

The pathetic truth is that German measles is a very benign disease lasting only a few days in most patients. The only people at risk are unborn babies of mothers who catch the disease during early pregnancy, a very small percentage of people and not warranting the massive vaccination program that started in 1979. Even more ironic, pregnant mothers are even more likely to come down with rubella infection because of the known transmissability of the virus from inoculated people. SO, like so many things in science, the end result of this experimentation has made the situation potentially worse.

Some interesting questions arise:

(1) Aren't these the same people who gave us the Swine flu vaccine (paralysis), gamma globulin (AIDS and hepatitis) and polio vaccine (brain cancer)?

(2) Are these vaccines used in Russia and by other enemy governments?

(3) Can you, with this terrible record, trust any vaccine recommended by public "health" officials?

(4) Are there Epstein-Barr or other viral contaminants involved here?

(5) Has anyone bothered to check? As Dr. Peyton Rous said in 1935: "Since what one thinks determines what one does in research, it is well to think something." What they should be thinking is, which virus is it this time and how did it get there.

(6) The most important question: Are all these young people dragging themselves around from doctor to doctor, looking for a cure for their fatigue, eventually going to get cancer, like many other victims of public health medicine?

A possible answer to that last question: Some experts suspect that the chronic fatigue syndrome, being spread through the German measles vaccine, is actually HBLV, Human B-cell leukemia virus. The presence of this deadly infectious cancer has increased over 200 percent in California during the past ten years. HBLV in humans is morphologically identical to the African swine fever virus. Is this another genetically-engineered virus created by the Fifth Horseman of the Apocalypse—the retrovirologists?

Another example of immunization medicine is a recent experience m Chicago where adults of the Chicago Mercantile Exchange suffered a large mumps epidemic. Did these young adults contract mumps from having received the mumps vaccine earlier in life, or did they perhaps catch it from their mumps-vaccinated children? Experts have long theorized that vaccination programs may just change childhood diseases into adulthood diseases.

Jean Carper, again in her article in the **World Book Encyclopedia,** 1970, summarized her thoughts on rubella vaccination: "It is now likely that, for the first time in thousands of years, the next ever-predictable rubella epidemic will not occur in countries where inoculation programs were undertaken. When it comes time for the virus to go on its rampage of destruction, to emerge again, it will find hardly a friendly human cell to occupy. This time, science got there first."

The question is, first with what?

Unfortunately AIDS is a moving target and *mutates many times faster* than the influenza virus. With tens of millions of various genetic variations possible with the AIDS virus, and the reality that many genetic combinations are spreading at the same time, including some times as many as two or three or more genetic varieties in the same patient, it is obviously futile, foolhardy, extravagant and deceitful to pursue the mirage of vaccination.

Our third question was: "Does vaccination work?"

Let us first look at other modern day examples of the failure of vaccinations, Then we will, briefly, follow the entire sordid vaccination history to make a case for pursuing some more reasonable form of defense against AIDS.

The most impressive application of vaccine inoculation in the history of medical science took place in Viet Nam between 1960 and 1972. In just the last four years of the Viet Nam War more than 17 million vaccinations were given against plague, which is endemic in Viet Nam.

Even in the face of extensive pesticide dusting to kill fleas, the effect on the incidence of plague was essentially zero. Between 1965 and 1970 over 25 thousand plague cases were reported in South Viet Nam, and the total was believed to be about 250,000 cases. It would appear that the vaccine, assuming that the pesticide program was somewhat successful, made the situation worse.

In July of 1947, a laboratory worker in Johannesburg, South Africa, came down with plague. He had received many injections of the plague-attenuated vaccine and the last shot only two weeks before his illness. He acquired pneumonic plague and was dead in four days.

Because of the extreme seriousness of plague in Fukin Province, northeast of Hong Kong, the populace was intensely vaccinated with plague vaccine, over 41 thousand doses. With the administration of the vaccine the situation got rapidly worse, and the yearly count went from 626 in 1941 to 5000 in 1943 and 7000 cases two years later.

In 1959 a laboratory chemist at the Ft. Detrick, Maryland, bio-chemical laboratory contracted plague. He had been adequately vaccinated, including receiving booster shots. He was one of the lucky ones to survive the plague—and the immunization.

A 21-year-old soldier stationed at Ft. Worth, Texas, had recently been transferred from Viet Nam. The army doctors first mis-diagnosed this case as "incarcerated hernia" and then later as "lymphoma." Two weeks later, miraculously, he was still alive, although infected with plague, and was finally diagnosed as such. Having been in Viet Nam, he had been "adequately vaccinated" with the plague vaccine. There are many, many instances of plague infection following "adequate" vaccination, indicating beyond a doubt that the immunization does not work.

The hepatitis-B immunization, also used by the armed forces, and for which Dr. Wolf Szmuness has received so much acclaim, is now seen to be of very limited value, if of any value at all.

The whole theory of immunization against disease is rooted in a belief in the immunity conferred by a non-fatal attack of the disease. Although some immunity does appear to be effective in some people, the results with artificial immunization have been too spotty to justify the wide degree of acceptance immunization shots have received.

Edward Jenner, who bought his medical degree for 15 pounds, and then stole the cowpox vaccination idea from a simple Welch farmer by the name of Benjamin Jesty, was unwittingly accepting the ancient Indian rite of subjecting people to an artificially induced attack of cowpox to propitiate Sheetula-Mata, the goddess of pox torment.

Jenner was a busybody with no medical education, no medical experience and a reckless disregard for the safety of his patients. Jenner, who had a very vivid imagination' held that "genuine" cowpox came from the "grease" of horses. He came to this momentous opinion by observing that horses had a skin condition that also produced blisters like cowpox.

He proceeded to prove his discovery by vaccinating a child with horse grease, taking it from the horse's hocks. He did indeed produce some handsome blisters on the child, and the child promptly died. This same type of helter-skelter logic led him to inoculate cows' teats with horse grease in an attempt to prove that the cowpox and the horse grease pox were the same.

Following Jenner's lead, that cowpox, horsepox and human smallpox were all the same, a Dr. Babcock pro-

ceeded to make a vaccine which was produced by injecting human smallpox into the udder surfaces of cows. He
bragged that his concoction had been used for 40 years
and had achieved great popularity in Brighton, England.
Doctors at Attleborough, Massachusetts, inoculated citizens with this cow-grown smallpox and disaster followed. There was an epidemic of smallpox, panic and a
suspension of the vaccination program.[14]

The concept of immunizing people against human diseases by using animal viruses is totally against the basic
rules of virology. The species barrier has always protected
man from most animal viruses. When one injects this foreign animal protein into a human there is certainly an immune response which is reflected in the blood. But this
immune response is to the foreign animal protein and not
to the human disease. It is highly unlikely, therefore, that
any protection is afforded by this process.

The value of cowpox as a protection against smallpox
may now be judged apart from the fanciful doctrine of
"cowpox is smallpox and smallpox is cowpox." It has
been put to a test extending over 180 years and it is now
possible to judge it on the basis of modern science. The
besetting fallacy of all vaccination logic is that of *post hoc
ergo propter hoc* (B follows A, therefore A caused B).

From the earliest period of its history in Europe, smallpox has had its seasons of quickening or revival, with
long periods of quiescence. During the early years of the
19th century there was a marked remission of the epidemic outbursts of the disease in most parts of Europe.
The amount of vaccination during these years was incon-
sequential. It is important to bear in mind the overall pe-
riodic exacerbation and dormancy, which makes it
extremely difficult to assess cause and effect. As Dr.
Creighton stated in the ninth edition of the **Encyclopedia**

---

14 *Boston Medical and Surgical Journal*, 1860, p. 77.

Brittanica, "Inoculation almost certainly interferred with the natural tendency of smallpox as a foreign pestilence to die out." Dr. Creighton concluded: "Absolute cessation of smallpox would have no more necessary connection with almost universal vaccination than the alternating quiescence and recrudescence of epidemics have been connected with each new act of Parliament."

The statistics of the 19th century clearly bear out this severe appraisal of smallpox vaccination by Dr. Creighton. At the Eastern Metropolitan Hospital, Homerton, England, there were between 1871 and 1878 6533 admissions for smallpox of which 4283 had been vaccinated. Only 1477 of the smallpox victims were unvaccinated.

In Bavaria in 1871, there was a devastating epidemic of smallpox. Thirty thousand of those infected had been vaccinated—95.7 percent of the cases. There is a question as to whether the smallpox contracted by someone vaccinated is more or less likely to cause death following infection. The figures from Bavaria are again quite startling. In the 1871 epidemic there were 4000 deaths among vaccinated persons and only 790 deaths among the unvaccinated.

A further indictment against smallpox vaccination was the fate of people who were re-vaccinated. In Prussia in 1835 re-vaccination of school pupils at the age of 12 was an integral part of the vaccination law. Notwithstanding the fact that Prussia was the most re-vaccinated country in Europe, its mortality from smallpox in the epidemic of 1871 was by far the highest in northern Europe.

All German troops in that era were also re-vaccinated. They had a death rate of 60 percent from the disease. The Bavarian contingent of the German army, which was totally re-vaccinated, had a death rate five times that of the general population where re-vaccination was not generally done.

In the Europe of a hundred years ago, as today, those who refused vaccination were considered trouble-makers and a source of disease that endangered the entire community. Smallpox, for example, was said to start among them, gather force and then overwhelm even the vaccinated part of the population. Enquiry into the actual facts in Cologne in 1870 revealed that the first unvaccinated person who contracted smallpox was the 174th person to actually get the disease. In Liegnitz in 1871 the first unvaccinated person to contract the disease was number 225.

Also reflecting today's herd instinct and zealous attitudes toward immunization, parents in England after 1867 were severely penalized if they refused to have their children vaccinated. In 1880 some local government boards wanted to repeal the harsh penalties but, not surprisingly, the medical profession protested and the penalties, even to the point of seizing private property, were kept in place.

The assertion is that because many people have had a "one and only" attack of any specific disease, "auto protection" has thus been afforded them. That is surely no more scientific than the old Indian belief in the assuaging of the wrath of Sheetula-Mata. As Professor Alfred Russel Wallace says: "Very few people suffer from any special accident twice—a shipwreck, or railway or coach accident, or a house on fire; yet one of these accidents does not confer immunity against its happening a second time. We have taken it for granted that second attacks of smallpox, or any other zymotic disease, are of that degree of rarity as to prove some immunity or protection, indicates the incapacity for dealing with what is a purely statistical question."[15]

Dr. Alfred Salter recalled a doctor who was quite adamant about the effectiveness of immunization *even*

---

15 Alfred Russel Wallace, L.L.D., **The Wonderful Century**, chapter 18, p. 296.

though his daughter had recent) died after a third attack of Scarlet fever.

In my practice I know of a gentleman who has had recurrent herpes zoster (shingles) of the groin 25 times. In medical school we were taught that recurrence of shingles was rare.

In 1872 Dr. Charles Creighton, the most respected epidemiologist of his time, stated: "The zymotic diseases replace each other; and when one is rooted out it is apt to be replaced by others which ravage the human race indifferently whenever the conditions of a healthy life are wanting. They have this property in common with weeds and other forms of life; as one recedes another advances."

This is known as the Substitution Theory which holds that elimination of one disease only leads to having it replaced by another, if living conditions and general health are poor enough to encourage a new round of infectious disease. Dr. Creighton, in his History of Epidemics in Britain, suggests that plague of the 14th, 15th and 16th centuries was replaced by typhus fever and smallpox. Later on measles, which had been insignificant before the middle of the seventeenth century, began to replace the latter disease. Florence Nightingale made note of this interesting replacement of one disease by another.

A modern example of this replacement theory is the current situation in West Africa. That area has not seen cholera since the nineteenth century. Yet, in August, 1970, cholera literally exploded on the scene causing 150,000 cases and 20,000 deaths.

Louis Pasteur, the father of modern immunization, while not a complete charlatan like Edward Jenner, was described by his professors as a poor chemistry student. He had absolutely no training and experience in medicine. Yet he set out to conquer disease, save mankind and at the same time make himself immortal. He thus created a hundred years of havoc in medicine, but he indeed did become immortal.

Dr. Charles Creighton, writing in the Encyclopedia Brittanica of the late nineteenth century, called vaccination a "grotesque superstition." Dr. A. H. Caron of Paris declared that he had long since positively refused to vaccinate at any price.

Professor Adolph Vogt, Professor of Hygiene and Sanitary Statistics at the University of Berne from 1877 to 1894, supplied a mathematical demonstration that a person who had once undergone smallpox was *63 percent more liable to suffer from it again in a subsequent epidemic than a person who had never been a victim to it.* Vogt concluded: "All this justifies our maintaining that the theory of immunity by a previous attack of smallpox, whether the natural disease or the disease produced artificially, must be relegated to the realm of fiction."[16]

Vaccination was intensively practiced in England and Wales from 1853 and in fact, was made compulsory in that year. They were so strict it was ordered that evaders of vaccination would be prosecuted and punished. the result was a precipitous increase in smallpox in England and Wales. In 1857-59 there were 14,244 deaths from smallpox, in 1863-65 there were 20,059 deaths; in 1870-72 there were 44,840 deaths. During the last of these epidemics (1877) the population increased by nine percent and deaths from smallpox increased 123 percent.

After all army troops were extensively vaccinated in the Philippines in 1899 ("The entire command has been vaccinated at least four times since the appearance of the disease.") the result was a precipitous increase in fatalities from smallpox. In 1899, at the beginning of the vaccination there was a 29 percent fatality rate. By 1900 this had gone up to 45.9 percent fatality rate.

---

16 Ibid.

Professor Alfred Russel Wallace remarked on studies done on British army and navy troops in the late nineteenth century. After studying the extensively smallpox-vaccinated troops and the results between 1873 and 1894 he concluded:

"It is thus completely demonstrated that all the statements by which the public has been gulled for so many years as to the almost complete immunity of the revaccinated army and navy are absolutely false It is all what the Americans call 'bluff.' There is no immunity. They have *no* protection. When exposed to infection they *do* suffer as much as other populations, or even more. In the whole of the 19 years: 1878-1896 inclusive, unvaccinated Leicester (a town in England) had so few smallpox deaths that the registrar represents the average by the decimal point 0.01 per thousand population, equal to 10 per million, while for the 12 years there was less than one death per annum! Here we have *real* immunity, *real* protection; and it is obtained by attending to sanitation and isolation, coupled with the almost total neglect of vaccination. Neither army nor navy can show any such results as this." (All emphasis is in the original statement.)

The Philippine experience mentioned above is such a dramatic example of the futility, in fact the insanity of vaccination, that it should be described in a little more detail.

"The Philippines have experienced three smallpox epidemics since the United States first took over the islands, the first in 1905-1906, the second in 1907-1908, and the third and worst of all, the recent epidemic of 1918-1919. Before 1905 (with no systematic general vaccination) the case mortality was about 10 percent. In the 1905-1906 epidemic, with vaccination well started, the case mortality ranged from 25-50 percent in different parts of the islands. During the epidemic of 1918-1919, with the Philippines supposedly almost universally immunized against smallpox by vaccination, the case mortality averaged over 65 percent."[17]

Commissioner General Leonard Wood reported in 1921[18] that "not only has smallpox become more deadly in the Philippines, but, in addition, the statistics of the Philippine Health Service show that *there has been a steady increase in recent years in a number of preventable diseases, especial) typhoid, malaria and tuberculosis.*"

The highest mortality from smallpox, 65.3 percent, was in Manila, the capital, and the most thoroughly vaccinated place in the islands. The lowest percentage of mortality, 11 percent, was in Mindanao, where, owing to religious prejudices of the inhabitants, vaccination had not been practiced.

Medical authorities, being generally fanatical in their beliefs and their support of vaccination medicine, forced the people of Mindanao to take vaccinations after 1918. The result has been a dramatic increase in mortality from the disease to 25 percent from a previous 11 percent. General Leonard Wood commented: "In view of the fact that the sanitary engineers had probably done more in Manila to clean up the city and make it healthy than in any other part of the islands, there is every reason to believe that excessive vaccination *actually brought on the smallpox epidemic* in spite of the sanitary measures to promote health." (Emphasis added.)

Pasteur, always quick to see the commercial profit possibilities with one of his nostrums, announced that he had a cure for anthrax, the deadly disease of sheep (and humans). Pasteur sold his anthrax vaccine to Kachowka in southern Russia where it was administered to 4500

17 Philippine Health Service, 1919, p.78. and The Masonic Observer, 14 July, 1922.
18 Report of the Special Mission on Investigation to the Philippine Islands.

207

sheep. Thirty-six hundred of them promptly died. In another experiment in that country 4500 sheep were vaccinated, and 3700 died of anthrax. The anthrax "vaccine" was so bad and so deadly that the country of Hungary officially prohibited its use, it was denounced in Germany, and the English Board of Agriculture declined to recommend it.

Pasteur's rabies vaccine turned out to be equally disastrous, and as Professor Michael Peter complained: "Pasteur does not cure hydrophobia—he gives it!"

Even royalty was not safe from the needles of Louis Pasteur. King Alexander of Greece was bitten by a monkey. The king's doctors looked to the great Pasteur for help. The king was perfectly fine until he started receiving the Pasteurian rabies vaccine and took a sudden turn for the worse. He was vaccinated a number of times and continued to weaken and finally died.[19]

It was learned by more realistic, independent thinking physicians that the best treatment for rabies was no Pasteurian immunization and a series of atropine injections.

E. Douglas Hume comments on the commercialization of science which started with Pasteur, truly the father of commercial science:

"Pasteur's inoculations for hydrophobia (rabies) form part of a vast money-making system, in which the beneficiaries have no wish that any item should be discredited... Thus we find science dominated by commercialism... It is the era for the injection into the blood of matter of varying degrees of offensiveness, the era in which animal experimentation, vastly increased, has found its sequence in experiments on human beings, and the credulous and ignorant are everywhere at the mercy of the subcutaneous syringe

---

19 *London Daily Mail*, October 1920.

and thereby swell the monetary returns of the manu-facturers of vaccines and serum."[20]

If it were not for the current mad dash for an inocula-tion against AIDS, we would not go into so much detail concerning the history of immunization. But it is ex-tremely important for the American people to realize that this is an entirely futile effort that will only create more calamities instead of less, and more millionaires.

An even more astounding example of the total futility and disastrous effect of immunization is that experienced by the British during the Gallipoli Peninsular Campaign in Turkey and also in the Boer War in South Africa.[21]

Every man had been rigorously inoculated against typhoid and the results were utter disaster. The total number of troops killed and missing was 37,700. The total number sick from typhoid. even though inocu-lated, was 96,684!

"In short," comments Dr. Hadwan, "the total of disease and death in these modern days of serums and vaccines, with all their 'protecting' influences against microbes, was nearly six times greater the last six months of the Gallipoli disaster."

The Boers were not defeated by the British but by ty-phoid. As *The Vaccination Enquirer* of March 1917, page 36, put it "It looks more than probable that the doctors have been at their ancient practice of sowing with one hand the disease which they pretend to cure with the other, of course in all stupidity and good faith."

This sad story has been repeated with diphtheria, yel-low fever and with every other disease that Pasteur's nee-dles were supposed to have eliminated.

In 1975 the World Health Organization announced that smallpox had been eradicated from the earth.

---

20   Hume, **Beauchamp or Pasteur?**, Daniel Company, England.
21   Walter R. Hadwan, **Microbes and the War,** Whitehall, London.

Champaign parties were held all around and everyone congratulated themselves on this great achievement. Vaccination had proven itself to be the great medical wonder that chemist Pasteur said it would be. May we suggest a pause before congratulating ourselves on total elimination of the first of the diseases of man? Herbert Spencer once said "When once you interfere with the order of nature, there is no knowing where the results will end.

"Jenner and his disciples," Spencer said, "have assumed that when vaccine viruses pass through a patient's system he is safe, or comparatively safe, against smallpox, and that there the matter will end. I merely propose to show that there the matter does *not* end. Interference with the order of Nature has various consequences other than that counted upon. Some have been made known." Herbert Spencer was more right than he could ever have possibly imagened.

Spencer continues: "You cannot change the constitution in relation to one invading agent and leave it unchanged in regard to all other invading agents" (The substitution theory).

And this, perhaps the most compelling of Spencer's remarks on Jenner, Pasteur and immunization: "We have no means of measuring alterations and resisting power, hence they commonly pass unremarked. There are, however, evidences of a general relative debility period. Measles is a severer disease than it used to be, and deaths from it are very numerous. Influenza yields proof. Sixty years ago, when at long intervals an epidemic occurred, it seized but few, was not severe, and left no serious sequella; now it is permanently established, affects multitudes in extreme forms, and often leaves damaged constitutions. The disease is the same but there is less ability to withstand it."

Note that this was written before the great 1918 influenza epidemic that killed tens of millions of people throughout the world.

The World Health Organization, in "eradicating" smallpox has, as we have pointed out in a previous chapter, inundated the world with a far worse scourge—AIDS. But we doubt that the replacement has been complete and we forecast that smallpox will return.

A vaccination for AIDS? The whole endeavor is futile, dangerous and fraught with many medical complications even beyond the present AIDS epidemic, including the terrible possibility of further stimulating infectious cancers, neurological diseases and AIDS itself.

RECOMMENDED READING:

Dutton, **Worse Than the Disease,** Cambridge University Press, New York.

Hume, **Beauchamp or Pasteur?,** Lee Foundation for Nutritional Research, Milwaukee, Wisconsin 53201.

Chapter 10
AIDS and Youth

Once we start seeing AIDS cases in the 18-2+ year-old female population, we'll be behind the eight ball."

Thomas Quinn, M.D.
National Institute of Allergy
and Infectious Diseases

The news media and misguided teachers "educating" our children about AIDS are doing great harm. A new TV commercial tells kids after the Saturday morning cartoons: "AIDS can't be caught by sharing pencils or school books."

What about sharing water or food? What about sneezing and coughing? What about wrestling, biting, and kissing? What if the AIDS-infected child has tuberculosis, hepatitis or an incipient meningitis? Pencils? School books? That is a deadly and criminal misdirection of the child's attention from many very real dangers of "casual" association with AIDS-infected children.

While at a conference in Las Vegas, Nevada, Dr. Robert Strecker, an authority on AIDS, was talking to a school teacher who taught in the Las Vegas high school system. She told him a very interesting and frightening story about blood bank collection at one of the local schools. Three thousand units of blood had been collected from the students and .5 percent checked positive for AIDS.

One half of one percent does not sound like a lot, one in 200 students, but it's a great deal more than the one in 300, reported in a recent survey of college students. Keeping in mind that these college students with AIDS undoubtedly caught it while in high school, this difference would indicate that the college figure may be low and that AIDS will be even more rampant in colleges in the very near future.

It's interesting to note that this grim finding was not reported in the press, even the *local* press.

Neva Snell, assistant promotion manager for TV station WXEX, says, "Why not let them know it isn't something they have to be afraid of?" My God, where has this woman been?

Another "expert" said, "For young people to be talking to other young people saying you don't need to be afraid of a kid who has AIDS... is good."[1] The source of that pearl of wisdom was Holly Smith, an officer in the San Francisco AIDS Foundation. Don't believe anything you read about AIDS that comes out of San Francisco.

The state of Georgia illustrates the pervasive and pernicious influence that homosexuals have on AIDS public school policy. The Board of Education wanted to require AIDS-infected children to be taught at home and to dismiss teachers with the disease. But that would have run counter to the recommendations of the Georgia Task Force on AIDS. The Task Force is greatly influenced by the most AIDS-infected group—the homosexuals. The school boards, manipulated by a special interest group, are playing Russian roulette with your children.

Everyone read about the bubble AIDS child in Tampa, Florida, a pathetic situation where the mother is insisting that her *mentally retarded* child with AIDS attend regular school. A federal judge (Judges are one of the great menaces to our society, as Thomas Jefferson clearly recognized) has ordered that the child attend class in a plastic

---

1   *Walls Street Journal*. March 18,1987.

213

bubble "until she becomes toilet-trained and stops sucking her fingers."[2]

One parent, obviously more intelligent than the judge, said: "There's too much unknown to say AIDS is not a communicable disease." That's right on target and she probably doesn't even have a Ph.D.

A heavy gun, a professor of allergy from the University of South Florida, was brought in to soothe the parents. "Can you guarantee that the child will not infect our children?" a parent asked.

"No, I can't guarantee, but I can give you the medical information. A person walking around with the disease doesn't send it out like missiles."

The infected child can send out, "like missiles," many things including Q-fever, Tuberculosis, yeast, and a host of exceedingly dangerous viruses. You blend a dumb judge with a dumb doctor and you've got another dangerous missile.

Even more preposterous is the situation in Bibb County, Georgia. AIDS-infected children are put into classes heretofore reserved for gifted children, thereby exposing the county's gifted children to an even higher probability of contracting AIDS! Ask your school board if they are planning to place your child next to a sneezing, coughing, AIDS-infected child. If so, get him out of there. Find a private school that is not run by politicians.

Buried on page 14 of the March 1, 1987 *Atlanta Constitution* was an alarming statistic that the paper should have put on page one. It was a report on proposed AIDS instruction in Georgia schools. The statistic was this: In three months the number of AIDS-infected children in the state of Georgia had risen from three to 10. Doesn't sound like much does it, only seven more cases. But think of it in terms of compounded interest and what do you get?

2   AP, 8/25/88.

You get a holocaust if the trend holds true, that is what you get. If the rate of infection goes up 200 percent every three months, in a year and a half you will have about 3,000 dying children in the state of Georgia alone.

Sometimes students are ahead of the faculty. At the Citadel military college in Charleston, S.C., applicants are now screened for AIDS. The students want to go further. They say it defeats the school's purpose of an AIDS-free campus not to test *all* students *and* faculty members.

Child prostitution is contributing greatly to the international AIDS problem. Girls in their pre-teens and early teens in many countries can make five to 10 times more money than an adult prostitute. In Paris 5000 boys and 3000 girls work as prostitutes, and in Latin America a 12-yearold child can make 10 times as much money as an adult can make working in a factory.[3]

Recent studies have shown that 40 percent or more of teenagers are sexually active at the age of 14. One out of seven teenagers, which means two and a half million, have some form of venereal disease. Half a million have gonorrhea and 30 percent or more have Chlamydia. The figure for Chlamydia may be much higher.

The present number of teenagers who have active AIDS (200) is comparable to the number of homosexuals who had AIDS just six years ago. The problem complicating the situation with teenagers is that teenagers live longer than infected adults and develop the disease much slower. Three different studies have shown this. Longer incubation means a longer period of time to infect their peers.[4]

The schools, following the lead of Washington "experts" like Surgeon General C.E. Koop, are continuing to

3 *Christianity Today,* date unknown.
4 *AIDS Protection,* September, 1988, Vol. 2, No. 5.

give students advice based on unproven and often incorrect assertions. One student stated that she would not go barefoot this summer "because I'm afraid I could catch AIDS if I have a cut on my foot and step on spit from someone who has it."[5] Someone described as a "public health expert" by the *Atlanta Constitution* told her that "she has nothing to worry about" because the virus "just lives a few hours outside the body." This is *absolutely false* and reflective of the level of incompetence in most public health departments. Saliva is a *common source* of the AIDS virus and getting it on a cut would be a highly efficient way of contracting the disease.

A senior student asked, "Is it true that one in four of the high school kids who go to Florida over spring break will come back with AIDS?" The *Atlanta Constitution* editorializes: "The question shows the way false rumors spread about the disease sweeping through the student community."

The correct answer would have been: *No one knows,* because the incubation period may be as long as seven or even 10 years and at the present time we have *no idea* how many students are infected with the AIDS virus. We do know that a very high percentage of students at the college level carry at least one venereal disease. This makes them far more vulnerable to AIDS infection.

In spite of the AIDS plague, 40 percent of college women and 61 percent of college men engage in "recreational sex."[6] It is estimated that 30 percent of college girls have the venereal disease, chlamydia. That is only one of nine venereal or sex-associated diseases we

---

5 *Atlanta Constitution,* 3/24/88.
6 *Playboy,* 9/88.

are now dealing with.* One in seven of our youth currently has a sexually transmitted disease.[7] *How many of these students have AIDS?*

Twenty years ago we were assured that sex education would make for less venereal disease, a less neurotic world, and fewer teen pregnancies. I said then that it would *not* stop sexual promiscuity, would *increase* illegitimate pregnancies and would probably lead to an epidemic of V.D. among our young people. A generation later we have the highest teen pregnancy rate in the Western world and venereal disease is rampant among our youth.

The high priestess of sex education has always been Mary Calderone. I have been an implacable enemy of her corrupting "sex education" schemes for 25 years and have never hesitated to say so loudly and publicly. She now admits that sex education will not stop AIDS.[8] She says Americans are "addicted" to sex. Calderone, through her "how to do it" classes on sex, is primarily responsible for that addiction, but she *blames the parents.*

Joann Dale complained about the sex education given her child at a Fairfax County school. She told legislators that her daughter's seventh and eighth grade classes discussed practices such as anal sex, oral sex, beastiality and the methodology of male homosexuality and lesbian behavior. Children were told: "Your parents are from an-

---

* Trichomoniasis, chlamydia, herpes, genital warts, syphilis, gonorrhea, AIDS, amoebiasis and other intestinal parasites and hepatitis. There are two other particularly disgusting venereal diseases called granuloma inguinale and granuloma venerium which will probably make a comeback, especially in the homosexual population. Although these are not all technically venereal ("sexually transmitted") diseases, many of them are transmitted by close contact. Sex education has been very productive.

7 Ibid.
8 Newsweek, 9/24/86.

217

other generation and they wouldn't understand, because they are living in the dark ages."[9]

Because of the sexual promiscuity of our young people, AIDS will spread like the plague through our youth. The answer of the professional educators: more sex education. It makes about as much sense as teaching kids how to use needles "safely" and snort cocaine in order to reduce drug addiction. Sex education in the schools was a stupid idea. Now we're going to pay for it through the devastation of our children.

America's colleges report an intense interest in the AIDS epidemic, with courses always filled, but it has little impact on the sexual behavior of college students. They seem to *underestimate the crossover* among homosexuals, bisexuals and I.V. drug users. "After all," the girls think, "if he's attracted to me, obviously he isn't homosexual and if he were bisexual I could tell."

This is a *fatal error* that will lead to a dramatic increase in AIDS in the early 1990's *among our young science and business elite.*

What can you do for your children, the ones who will have to rebuild this nation? Take them out of school and teach them at home. The school system has been permissive about homosexuals and "alternate lifestyles" and has taught our children how to fornicate. The system is greatly responsible for the mess we are in. Unless you can find an extremely strict Victorian-type of school, such as a Jewish, Catholic, or Protestant institution that doesn't teach sex, you're going to have to teach your children at home.

We may have to write off most of a generation, just watch them die. But the younger ones can be saved by a return to pioneer-type personal responsibility and a strict morality. Look at your six-year-old. Is the government going to solve this problem? Are the doctors? Do you have a choice?

---

9   *AIDS Protection*, September, 1988, Vol. 2, No. 5.

But a caveat on the Catholic schools: 50 percent of priests are reported to be homosexual.[10] Maybe some sex education is worse than others.

But the Protestant churches are, if anything, even more influenced by the homosexual movement. Fr. Enrique Rueda in his exhaustive study, **The Homosexual Network,**[11] said:

"The reader is cautioned, however, not to conclude that the Roman Catholic Church has been chosen as the most 'homosexualized' church in the United States. Although within the Protestant tradition–using this word in its broadest sense–are found the clearest examples of rejection of homosexual behavior and even of the homosexual condition itself in fundamentalist preachers, mainline Protestant denominations are notorious for their willingness to compromise with the homosexual movement. For each example offered that shows elements within the Roman Catholic Church to be at the disposal of the homosexual cause, there are examples within Protestant denominations that show a far greater willingness to cooperate with the homosexual movement, even at the highest levels of authority."

The point is, you can't rely on schools and churches. You can't rely on the government or doctors to solve this problem. This is a family problem–which is what it has always been. We must have the courage to severely discipline our young. We must reassert control over our children so that the next generation can survive this holocaust.

Teen AIDS

"He looks about 17. Barefoot, dirty, he stumbles over to a garbage can and picks out bits of thrown-away french fries from under a crumpled *New York Times.*

---

10   *Wall Street Journal,* 2/19/87, pp 1.
11   The Davin Adair Co., Old Greenwich, Conn., 1982.

The purple lesions characteristic of Kaposi's sarcoma blotch his forehead and brows." The picture of teen AIDS in the big city.[12]

Dr. J.W. Curran of the CDC estimated in April that there were 7,000 AIDS-infected children between the ages of 10 and 19. In less than six months, he reports, there may be "thousands more."

These children are spreading AIDS on a daily basis. Most of them are involved in prostitution, and when they go home they take their AIDS with them. The potential for spread among our sexually-obsessed teenagers (thanks in part to sex education, the media and an indifferent home life) is enormous and it's happening.

How many of our children are AIDS positive? Nobody knows because nobody is testing. The rate maybe sky-rocketing, but under the current head-in-sand policies of federal, state and county health departments, we won't know for five to 10 years–when they start dying. Teen AIDS is a ticking time bomb.

There was a lot of press a few months ago about the tragic case of a young boy contracting AIDS from a blood transfusion. The publicity concerned his being denied the right to attend school with his peers. The courts forced the school to take him back. He would be especially vulnerable if another child, with whom he had close association, had been recently vaccinated. The AIDS-infected child could die from an overwhelming case of measles, chicken pox or mumps encephalitis caught from the recently vaccinated child. This is another example of how the medical bureaucrats and the courts are obsessed with rights rather than common sense.

In all the publicity there was never a word about the fact that the child with AIDS was being put at great risk.

12 *Medical Trib.*, August 26,1987.

In a crowded school environment he is constantly exposed to all of the childhood diseases, from measles to mumps, any one of which could kill him.

Teen AIDS will soon shock America into the reality of the AIDS pandemic. *Sixty-one percent of teen AIDS in New York City is among heterosexuals.* Sex education has led to promiscuity which will destroy our youth through AIDS. We are now approaching the end result of this "education"–skyrocketing venereal disease and tens of thousands of young Americans dying of AIDS.

Supporting this view, Dr. Donald Burke, Walter Reed Army Hospital, says AIDS will become more common among teenagers in the near future.[13]

The CDC has advised hospitals that extreme caution should be exercised around AIDS patients. Masks and gloves should be worn, clean with bleach, etc. Yet children are being forced to go to school with AIDS patients even if they have a cough or runny nose, and no one has suggested masks and gloves for *them.*

In the face of this biological warfare how much longer are the American people going to put up with General Koop's condomania, "safe sodomy," "sex education" and "confidentiality?" Koop is starting to back off. In a recent television interview he said, "I'm not particularly proud of my role in this condom business."

How long does it take to educate a 12-year-old about sex today? It takes about 15 seconds. You tell him: "If you do naughty things with your pee-pee you are going to die." It's as simple as that. Tell the sex expert at the school to buzz off. You don't want your children to know how to "avoid pregnancy," "practice safe sex" and indulge in "alternative life styles." Instructions in orgasm and anatomy, with or without condoms, is only feeding fuel to the AIDS bonfire.

---

13 *New England Journal of Medicine,* 317:131,1987.

It's interesting to see the handwringing start. Mainstream, morally neutral publications such as People Magazine are beginning to take a second look at television, music and music videos.

In a feature article on teen sex, *People* Magazine revealed some of this agonizing re-appraisal: "How could we expect (the teens) to 'be careful' when, by the estimate of one family planning group, there were 20,000 instances of 'suggested sexual intercourse' in 1986's TV programing?"

People Magazine says that sex education has failed. Actually it hasn't failed. Every screwball liberal, and those to the left of him, knew what they were promoting. They were hell-bent for sex education. The result has been exactly what was planned: 3,000 teen pregnancies per day and corruption of our youth.

Wouldn't it be ironic if the godless Russians and other communist countries, because of their Victorian attitude toward sex and their severe repression of homosexuality, escaped most of the ravages of the AIDS epidemic and took us over by simply walking across the Mexican border?

The CDC has asked for $21.7 million for "AIDS education." What a farce. The adult and teen populations already know:

1) How the disease is spread (or at least as much as anyone knows, including the scientists).

2) That condoms may prevent AIDS (or may not).

3) That contraceptive cream kills the AIDS virus.

Our children are getting education on AIDS and sex, but they're not getting the education they need. What they need to be told is:

1) Promiscuous sex, in fact any sex outside of wedlock, is very dangerous.

2) We don't know with certainty how AIDS is spread.

3) It is dangerous to associate with AIDS-infected people.

4) The AIDS-infected carry many other dangerous and highly communicable diseases.

5) The disease is rapidly spreading through our youth.

6) You cannot always recognize homosexuals and especially bi-sexuals who are transferring the disease from the homosexual community to the heterosexuals.

7) Drugs and AIDS are closely related. Drugs lead to a lessening of inhibitions which leads to promiscuous sex which leads to AIDS.

8) They must understand that with the long incubation period between acquiring the disease and having a positive test means that at this point we do not know who has AIDS and who does not. Because of this uncertainty, the only way to avoid AIDS is to avoid sexual contact, and even casual contact as much as possible, with AIDS-infected persons.

Chapter 11
The Arthropod Conspiracy

Dr. Mark Whiteside of the Institute of Tropical Medicine in Miami says that he doesn't buy the argument that AIDS is only transmitted through sexual contact and by blood. Whiteside said, "Every major epidemic in history has been linked to environmental factors."[1] With cholera and typhoid it was water. With tuberculosis it was aerosol spray (coughing and sneezing) and fomites (towels, handkerchiefs, dishes, etc.). Smallpox was transmitted by fomites and food. *With all other epidemics in history— yellow fever, denge fever, plague, malaria, typhus —insects were the vector.*

Whiteside and Dr. Caroline MacLeod, also of the Institute of Tropical Medicine, are suing the government, claiming that CDC officials are suppressing information that might confirm the insect-trasmission of the AIDS virus.

"Contrary to the myths perpetuated by the federal Centers For Disease Control," they said, "AIDS is a blood-transmitted disease that satisfies none of the classic criteria for a strictly sexually-transmitted disease. The campaign for safe sex/no sex and clean needles/no needles is necessary but insufficient to control this epidemic. *Neglecting the increasing) obvious environmental links to AIDS will lead to disaster."* The "environmental links" that Whiteside and MacLeod are referring to is the possibility of AIDS being transmitted by mosquitoes.

"Environmental disease is not 'frightening' in the sense that more can be done about it once it is recognized," they

---

1 *Discover*, December 1985.

added. "There is only so much you can do about people having sex. The American people can handle the truth about AIDS. *They won 't tolerate a cover-up as to the true causes and transmission of AIDS.* The issue of environmental factors and AIDS is more political and economic than scientific. This concept was well illustrated by your attempts to discredit insect transmission of AIDS in the absence of scientific data.

"If the U.S. public can be hoodwinked into believing that AIDS can be explained solely on the basis of 'poor people having too much sex,' then they won't spend the money to clean up the worst slums or develop necessary programs to control AIDS. Environmental improvements must go hand-in-hand with education if any program is to be successful. In the long run, programs that prevent disease will save billions of dollars since treatment is an endless drain on resources."[2]

Their attorney, Mark Leeds, added: "The defendant (the U.S. government) is withholding information about half the people found to have AIDS (in the Belle Glade study). There is no way to check on the accuracy when they are withholding so much information."[3]

MacLeod was interviewed on Good Morning America. Opposing her was Dr. Gary Noble. Dr. Noble said that the children of Belle Glade, Florida, where AIDS is an epidemic, had been checked and they had found no children carrying the antibody for AIDS.

Dr. MacLeod countered with an observation that the testing was poorly done and unreliable. She also pointed out that 40 percent of the AIDS-infected children of Africa have AIDS-Dee mothers. So where did they get AIDS? Insects in Central Africa are heavily infected with the virus. She could also have pointed out that a study in Zaire re-

---

2   *The New Federalist,* 77/88.
3   *Vindicator,* 7/27/88.

vealed that children with malaria were several times more likely to test positive for AIDS. There is only one way to get malaria and that's through mosquito bites.

The Pasteur Institute did a study a few years ago in which mosquitoes in Africa were found not to carry the AIDS virus. This year a repeat investigation revealed that 30 percent of mosquitoes tested in Africa are infected with the AIDS virus.

Joan Lunden asked Dr. Noble if he would state categorically that you can't catch AIDS from mosquitoes. He equivocated.

Sources within the CDC informed us that a CDC hit man, Dr. Castro, was sent to Florida in an attempt to suppress the mosquito story and to discredit Whiteside and MacLeod. He was fairly successful but we haven't heard the end of this mosquito business. Dr. Bernard Greenberg of the University of Illinois says the CDC "is not taking blood-sucking insects seriously."

Dr. Marvin J. Blazer of the VA Medical Center in Denver agrees with Dr. Whiteside:

"I believe that several pieces of information suggest a possible role for insect-borne spread in the tropics.. 50 of 75 serum samples collected from healthy children in the West Nile region of Uganda... had antibody to (AIDS)." He points out that heterosexual or homosexual transmission is unlikely in these children.

Blazer added that the distribution of antibodies for the HIV virus in Africa is known to be focal, i.e., localized to certain geographical areas. Clearly diseases that are spread strictly by the venereal method would not be choosy about their geography. The only known explanation for this focal or geographic spread would be some sort of insect with a limited range of activity. In Venezuela it was found that a significantly higher percentage of persons with malaria also had antibodies to

AIDS (25 percent). The general population had only a one percent infection rate.[4]

Dr. Jean-Claude Chermann of the Pasteur Institute has reported finding the DNA of the AIDS virus in nearly every African insect that he has studied that has had contact with humans. "These data," he said, "suggest that insects could be a reservoir or a vector for the AIDS virus."[5]

Perhaps even more startling and worrisome is the fact that Chermann found 30 percent of the insects tested contained the AIDS virus whereas in most insect-borne diseases *only three percent of insects are found to be infected.* In other words, the AIDS virus is *10 times* more concentrated in these insects than the concentration generally considered necessary for insect-transmission of disease.

Dr. William Haseltine, Dana Farber Cancer Institute, said, "AIDS may, in fact, be transmissible by... mosquito bites."

Dr. James Slaff, National Cancer Institute, said: "There is epidemiological evidence both in America and in Africa that mosquitoes have the potential to transmit the (AIDS) virus."

Dr. Neovyn Greaves of the University of London Institute for Cancer Research, flying in the face of most of the "expert opinion" around the world: "We've looked at the contrary evidence of sexual transmission and blood transfusion *and concluded that the evidence is rather weak.*"[6]

It has been proven conclusively that the AIDS virus can be found in mosquitoes 48 hours after digesting infected blood. Thousands of HIV particles can be found in one single white blood cell but only a hundred or so particles of virus are necessary to successfully infect a chimpanzee experimentally.[7] *The AIDS virus can be found in all*

---

4 Volsky, et. al. NEJM, Part 6, 1986.
5 Becker, ct. al. C.R, Academy of Science, Paris.
6 *AP*, Release 26, September 1986.
7 Hu, et. al. *Nature*, 328:721-723, 1987.

layers of the skin. The virus of AIDS can easily travel the feeding tube of a mosquito and enter a human being fed upon. Eighty different species of RNA virus are known to be transmitted to humans by mosquitoes and other bloodsucking insects.[8]

A friend went to donate blood at her local bank and they asked her if she had had any acupuncture treatments lately. Her question to me: "If they are worried about acupuncture needles transmitting AIDS why aren't they worried about mosquitoes?"

Answer: Some people are worried about mosquitoes in spite of reassurances from the CDC. A research team from the National Institute of Health reports that the AIDS virus can "ride as passenger" on the bloodsucking mosquito.[9]

Any living creature can get an AIDS-like disease. Cattle, sheep, pigs, cats, dolphins, chickens, bacteria like those in your intestine, parasites like malaria and insects are all susceptible to these lethal viruses. Even other viruses can "get" AIDS by a method called recombination.

When the Centers for Disease Control (CDC) and the Surgeon General, Dr. C.E. Koop, tell you that "you can't get AIDS from mosquitoes" they are dealing in half truth. Which means they are dealing in a half lie. "Mosquito" hardly covers the field of arthropod taxonomy. Maybe mosquitoes, a member of the arthropod family of insects, don't carry AIDS. But what about head lice, ticks, bed bugs, fleas, kissing bugs, and biting flies as possible AIDS carriers?

Viruses carried by these arthropod insects (arthropod means having joints) are called arboviruses which is a shortened version of arthropod-borne viruses. There are

---

8 Sanford, **Harrison's Principles of Internal Medicine,** 1977, 8th edition.
9 *Time,* July 13, 1987, pp.56.

500 identified arboviruses and 100 of these have already been associated with disease in man, many of them fatal.

An interesting possibility for AIDS transmission is the African swine fever virus, (ASF). The ASF virus looks like this:

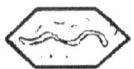

A deadly infectious cancer now seen in man, called HBLV (human B-lymphotrophic virus) looks like this:

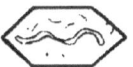

Do you detect a slight resemblance? An important rule in virology is that if two virus particles look the same then they are the same.[10]

If you have a history of Epstein Barr (E.B.V.) infection you'd better shun pigs and pig ticks. The EB virus makes your B-lymphocytes permissive to HBLV infection.[11] E.B.V. opens the door, so to speak, to this AIDS variant.

Dr. Jane Teas of Harvard was the first scientist to point a finger at swine. She wondered if pigs in Belle Glade were carrying ticks that were transmitting AIDS to pigs and people. She had done studies at Boston University and found that 10 of 21 AIDS patients were positive for ASF vius.[12] The CDC said that they could not duplicate her work.

The CDC is not good at duplicating studies that they don't want the public to know about. Remember that you are dealing with "political science," the ultimate oxymoron, when reading reports from the CDC. They sabotage their own experiments. You can imagine what they would do to someone like Teas who is not following the party line.

---

10 Joklik, **Virology**, 2nd Edition.
11 *Brit Med. J.*, 294:938-39,1987.
12 *The Atlantic Monthly*, September, 19B7. The entire article on insects and AIDS is highly recommended.

I called the CDC and asked to speak to someone in the virology department. A cold voice came on the line: "Yes?" I told this female voice, name unknown, that I was Dr. Douglass and I was very interested in AIDS. I wondered about the relationship between AIDS and the African swine ever vlrus.

"I've never heard of it," she replied.

"Oh. (Pause in disbelief.) Do you mean you have never heard of the relationship or you've never heard of the virus?"

"Never heard of the virus–why don't you check the literature. That would be my suggestion." I could feel her eagerness to hang up.

"Fine, would you like copies of what I come up with?" No response, another awkward pause. "Well, thank you."

"You're welcome, good-bye." Click.

I have been very hard on the CDC. Maybe I flatter myself, but I got the feeling from the outset of our conversation that I was considered an unfriendly alien. Next time I won't identify myself.

Allow me to belabor the point. Can you imagine a scientist in the virology department of the Centers for Disease Control, the agency that is assigned the job of protecting as from infectious disease, not having heard of the African swine fever virus? I've heard of it. I even know what it looks like. *You* now know what it looks like. Dr. Jane Teas of Harvard knows about it. The Atlantic Month. magazine and all of its tens of thousands of readers know about it. Even African swine know about it. Everybody except Doctor Whatever-her-name-is at the CDC knows about it.

Teas called the University of Miami and asked if there were many pigs in Belle Glade. The poor people were getting AIDS in Belle Glade. Poor people often keeps pigs. You don't see many pigs at *1600 Pennsylvania Avenue or Number 10 Downing Street.*

"Nope, no pigs–lots of chickens," she was told. Dr. Teas knows that you have to check everything. She went to Belle Glade and the place was crawling with swine. In fact it was crawling with dying swine. One farmer said in classic understatement, "We have a problem with hogs."

The "problem" is probably African swine fever and Belle Glade's problem may be HBLV-induced AIDS-like disease from hogs to ticks to man.

Although Dr. Teas' theory has not been accepted by the medical bureaucrats it makes more sense than any explanation the CDC has come up with. The world's most eminent specialist in retrovirology, Dr. Robert Shope, said, "To hypothesize that AIDS might be transmitted by flies or other insects is perfectly logical and within the realm of possibility."[13]

A Brazilian expert, Dr. Ricardo Veronesi, said that he is "absolutely convinced" that mosquitoes will become involved in AIDS transmission in Brazil.[14]

Dr. MacLeod: "There are going to be dozens of viral epidemics in the next 15 years" and Dr. Whiteside made this grim statement: "If you have a few arboviruses plus AIDS, it's all over."

Because of the clear and present danger from mosquitoes, there should be an all out attack on mosquitoes in the United States, using DDT or whatever other insecticide that is not toxic to man and animals. Doing this *now* could save millions of lives later.

---

13 Ibid.
14 *The Washington Times*, 7/2/87.

Chapter 12
The Virology of AIDS

> *Those not familiar with biological terminology may wish to skip this chapter.*

The AIDS virus is called a retrovirus because it contains an enzyme called reverse transcriptase. This enzyme enables a virus, once it enters your cells, to inject its own genetic code directly into the genes of your cells, making *an irreversible bonding* of the victim's cells and the disease—a permanent relationship. Because of this remarkable capacity of the retroviruses, there will not be a cure for AIDS probably in our lifetime. Because of this deadly characteristic of the AIDS virus, the only hope for the human race would appear to be prevention rather than cure.

The AIDS virus is remarkable in many other ways. It wears a protective coat. It mutates at least 10 times faster than the cold virus, which in itself mutates rapidly. And, its most devastating feature, it destroys the immune system which is the very shield that man has depended upon through the ages to protect himself from infectious diseases. It is analogous to an incoming intercontinental ballistic missile which, as it approaches, knocks out the entire defense system of the nation before impact. It delivers its own one-two punch: destruction of the immune system which is followed by any number of a hundred different diseases and then death.

The AIDS virus is very distinctive and doesn't look like anything but one particular animal virus called bovine visna virus. It is almost certainly a laboratory recombinant organism composed of bovine leukemia virus and sheep visna virus.

It was a fateful day for the world when man learned how to take two separate viruses and introduce them into human tissue culture cells and thus produce a new form of life which is then virulent to humans rather than to the animals from which it came. Icelandic scientists were the first ones to actually grow an animal virus in human cells when they took the sheep visna virus and cultured it in cells from a human embryo in 1961. The technology grew rapidly, and now it's a simple matter to devise and alter almost any known animal virus and make it virulent to man.

One of the cardinal rules of virology is that if two viruses look alike, i.e. they have the same shape, design and size, then they are almost certainly the same virus, a very simple and easy to understand rule.[1] When the AIDS virus is isolated from a human and compared with the recombinant visna virus, it is obvious that they are identical. They are also identical in molecular weight, purple banding, gene codons, magnesium dependency and all the other criteria used to identify viruses.

A few drawings will help to fill in this important piece of the AIDS puzzle. This virus:

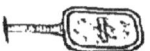

a virus of bacteria, (bugs have their troubles, too) doesn't look anything like a virus of ticks:

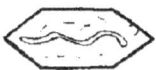

that's transmitted to pigs (and people), or this virus which is found in horses:

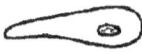

---

1   Joklik, **Virology**, second edition, p. 36.

The AIDS virus which "couldn't have come from animal viruses" is almost certainly a recombinant virus from fusing a cattle virus, bovine leukemia virus:

with sheep visna virus:

You combine the two in human tissue culture cells and you get bovine visna virus:

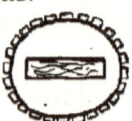

Now if you isolate the AIDS virus from an infected human it looks like this:

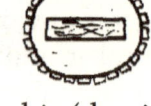

It doesn't look like this (the tick virus):

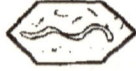

or *this* (the cattle virus):

it looks like this:

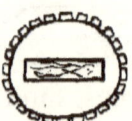

- the recombinant virus from cattle and sheep *and it's called AIDS*. You don't have to be a genius to understand this. Any properly instructed 10-year-old can understand it. For in stance, if you showed a 10-year-old one of these:

and then showed him one of these:

he would say that they are different. But he would quickly recognize the fact that this:

was like the first one and therefore was a rabbit. Very simple. But the virologists think that we are so simple-minded that we won't catch on to this. We are going to change that conception.

Even though some concede that AIDS may have come out of a laboratory, they feel that the epidemic was accidental. But an increasing number of scientists have concluded that it was a delib erate, carefully planned and well-executed biological invasion of the free world by Soviet and other eastern bloc scientists from the confines of the biological warfare laboratory at Fort Detrick, Maryland.

Nucleic acids are the building blocks of life. In the human cell the flow of information from your genes is from DNA to RNA and then to protein structure. It has always been considered impossible for the information to flow backwards (RNA to DNA). But retroviruses can do this. That's why they are called "retro." Retro stands for reverse transcriptase. Retroviruses contain this enzyme which enables the RNA virus to form a DNA copy of itself and then incorporate itself into your genes. It's part of your *permanent gene pool.* That's why there may be a treatment some day but probably never a cure.

An article by Stewart A. Arenson in 1972 entitled "Common Genetic Alterations of RNA Tumor Virus As Grown in Human Cells" revealed that the RNA tumor viruses when grown in human cells in a *laboratory* will incorporate into their own genes the human genes and therefore adapt to grow in humans, thereby causing infections in humans–a "species jump."

There is some evidence that the herpes virus is transmissible through condoms. *But* the AIDS virus *is smaller than the herpes virus.* The good news is that the virus of AIDS is *within* the lymphocytes and, because of their large size, the condom will block penetration—*unless broken* (which happens about 10 percent of the time).

The AIDS virus genes are not homologous with the genes of the monkey and they are incompatible with human genes. That means they don't "match up," so the virus didn't come from the monkey and it didn't come from man.

Last summer I watched "The Infiltrator," a high tech, sci-fi adventure story from CBS Summer Playhouse. It had the usual female-dominant heroine with a slightly bubble-headed male lead a la Bruce Willis, which is standard in late 20th century television. But the script had a remarkable (and accidental) corollary with today's science-gone-mad.

The snooty and all-business lady-scientist had invented a space probe that looked like the eyeball of a dinosaur with a hangover. It floated in air and was ready for the great trek into unknown galaxies.

But a strange thing happened on the way to Melmack. Her would-be boyfriend-scientist-flake, through the process of "teleportation," catapulted himself into her lab right through a steel door.

Well *that's* okay, but in the process of teleporting himself, complete with steaming clothes, he managed to incorporate the genes of the space probe into his body. The floating eyeball disappeared and became part of him. His genes and the probe's genes amalgamated into a new person. He became a monster and a killer.

Pretty wild, but no wilder or more terrifying than what is happening in biological science today. The mad scientists of the National Cancer Institute (NCI) and the World Health Organization (WHO) have actually created such biological freaks. They are known as AIDS victms.

It's unimaginable that scientists could have created in a retrovirology laboratory an agent that would infiltrate human cells and change these cells in such a way that they would *contain the genes of a cow and a sheep*–a new species created by man rather than God.

It sounds preposterous, but it is true. The African green monkey took the murder rap, *being fingered by the perpetrators of the crime*–the scientists in the subversive World Health Organization and their dupes in the National Cancer Institute, the National Institute of Health and the biological laboratories at Fort Detrick, Maryland.

The virologists injected bovine (cow) leukemia virus and sheep visna virus into human tissue cells called Hela cells. The result of this combination of two RNA retroviruses in human tissue cells was the formation of a "pro-virus" called bovine visna virus. This new genetic combination of viruses, half animal and half human, when given to humans, as it was in the great African smallpox vaccine program, causes AIDS.

Nature tends to eliminate variants. Anomalous creatures are either aborted or die soon after birth. How many cyclops do you see walking the streets? They are born occasionally, but seldom live. The few grotesquely deformed who survive after birth are usually sold to circuses, can't reproduce and die young. If there is ever a cure for AIDS, will these genetically-altered people be able to reproduce? I'm afraid the answer is yes because many AIDS-infected people have already had babies. Will the babies eventually reproduce?

Nature has never stood for the reproduction of freaks, no humans with the head of sheep. Nature likes order. But maybe with this genetic tinkering that has led to AIDS, man has succeeded in changing the rules of nature. (If the person next to you orders hay for dinner, be suspicious.)

Do we really want a cure for AIDS ? Do we want people, *carrying animal genes,* to reproduce? Don't pray for something unless you are sure you want it.

The retrovirologists can even splice plant genes into human tissue cultures and then inject that hybrid into humans. We would then have plant genes mixed into the human gene pool. The term cabbage-head may take on new meaning.

From 1911-1951 tissue cultures were only done in animal cells. Humans are humans and animals are animals. *The viruses grown in animal tissue cultures had never been grown in human tissue cultures. If you give the AIDS human virus to animals nothing happens.* Nature's "species barrier" has always protected animals from humans and humans from animals where retro-viruses are concerned. It was only after 1951, when human tissue cultures were developed, that it was possible to have a *fated contamination* and produce a lethal retrovirus for humans.

As early as 1970 WHO was growing these deadly viruses in human tissue cultures. *Cedric Mims, in 1981, said in a published article that there was a bovine virus contaminating the culture media of the WHO.* Was this an accident or a "non-accident?"

You can postulate that the AIDS virus "spontaneously mutated" to attack humans, but it's *very unlikely* that you would have a spontaneous mutation of a *whole family* of viruses to attack humans–HTLV-I, II, III (AIDS), IV, SV-40, STLV, ASFV, etc.

More bad news on AIDS comes from a federal research facility. It has been discovered that the virus can hide undetected in the bone marrow. "Latent viruses probably maintain a powerful reservoir in the bone marrow and thus can send infected cells through the body."[2]

A recent Army report reveals that the AIDS virus hides in certain cells called macrophages and *cannot be detected.* This means that many people thought free of AIDS, although they were in close contact with AIDS carriers, *may indeed be carrying the virus and spreading it to others.*

This finding gives a "painful message of uncertainty"[3] to epidemiologists as well as the rest of us because the carrier cells, the macrophages, go everywhere and can be "filled to bursting" with AIDS virus *and yet the body doesn't detect it.* Favorite hiding places are bone and brain.

Scientists have admitted that they have no idea how common these hidden cases are but they reassured the press that there is no cause for alarm because people at high risk of AIDS infection *"were asked"* (!) not to donate blood and because "they believe" most AIDS carriers carry detectable antibodies.[4]

But Dr. Monte S. Weltzer of Walter Reed Army Hospital admits that *"there is no way to gauge the proportion of high risk people who have AIDS infection yet negative antibody tests ...."*

The National Institute of Dental Research reported that saliva from three healthy men stopped AIDS from infecting blood cells.[5] Yet saliva in AIDS-infected persons will transmit the disease by biting. The anti-AIDS factor in saliva must be lost or overwhelmed when a person gets AIDS.

A report at the Stockholm conference on AIDS revealed that the outer envelope of the AIDS virus mutates

---

2 *Science News,* 3/7/88.
3 *New York Times,* 6/5/88.
4 Ibid.
5 *JADA,* 5/88.

very rapidly. This means that antibodies against one strain which would attack that particular envelope do not prevent infection against another strain. This is particularly relevant as some research presented at the conference showed that it is possible to isolate different strains of the virus from the same person at different times after infection. It was reported that the reason the killer T-cells might not destroy all the cells infected with the virus is because some of the infected cells hide "in immunologically privileged" sites such as bone and brain. T-cells cannot reach these sites, thus the virus can grow unmolested.

The research trying to develop a vaccine using the envelope proteins of the virus continues. Many experts feel this maybe very dangerous, because some scientists believe that the envelope protein is what actually causes the body to produce antibodies that cause the AIDS disease. Attempts to find a vaccine for any of the other AIDS-type of viruses found in sheep, goats and horses have been totally ineffectual *and in most cases the vaccines created cause the disease to become worse.*

The question arose at the meeting as to why some people among heterosexuals seem to catch the disease very quickly, whereas others do not. It is believed this may be because some people are "good transmitters" whereas others are not. Also some people may be infectious only at certain times, as in Hepatitis-B infection. Or their ability to infect others may vary with time, that is, a year from now the infected person may be far more infectious than he is at present.

One finding that goes against the current government information on AIDS is that the frequency of unprotected vaginal or anal intercourse did not seem to influence the risk of transmission. On the other hand, the researchers identified two cases of women who had become infected

with AIDS after only one reported act of sexual intercourse. This further strengthens the argument of Dr.
Robert Strecker, Dr. John Seale and myself that AIDS is
not a sexually transmitted disease, but is contracted only
incidentally through the sex act. Dr. Johnson, from the
Middlesex Hospital Medical School said, "The data on
heterosexual transmission presented at the conference
were consistent in that all the studies point to *wide variations in infectivity between individuals.*"

There are now six known varieties of the herpes virus.
The latest one, herpes-6, is believed to be a co-factor in
AIDS. It appears that a combination of the herpes-6 virus with the AIDS virus causes a lethal union with
rapid destruction of cells. It is believed that herpes-6 is
possibly involved also in chronic fatigue syndrome and
B-cell leukemm.[6]

Keeping the Players Straight:

HTLV-I   - T-cell leukemia
HTLV-II - Hairy cell leukemia
HTLV-III - **AIDS** (also called HIV)
HTLV-IV - **AIDS II** (HIV II)
HTLV-V - Mycosis fungoides leukemia and AIDS III

HTLV-I is now making headlines. The grim facts about
this genetically-engineered cattle virus, now infecting humans, are slowly coming out. (Truth by eye dropper as
the French say.)

• It can be carried by insects.
• It is highly communicable (a mother passed it to her
  two adult children, one of whom passed it to his two
  girl friends, one of whom passed it to her husband).
• There is no reliable test for it and it has contaminated
  our blood supply.

---

6   *Internal Medicine New,* 8/15-31/88.

• It may have a latency of 10 or more years. Which means that we will be facing a new wave of leukemia in the 1990's. It has, in fact, already started.

The fifth form of infectious leukemia was reported from Italy in December, 1987. It is called HTLV-V. It is "nique, according to Dr. Zah Salahuddin of the National Cancer Institute, in that it can go tvvo ways. It can cause either leukemia, like HTLV-I, or it can cause AIDS. (Some choice, like choosing between hanging and being shot).

A remarkable discovery, which has scientists baffled, concerns babies infected with AIDS from their mothers. Babies can be born with a quite different strain of HIV and, in fact, *a single infected cell can be found to harbor as many as seven genetic variations of the AIDS virus.*

New Scientist, 6/23/88, reports: "The current method—growing the virus through several generations and strains of cultured human cells—tends to select artificially for certain strains of AIDS that grow well in culture. Molecular biologists, therefore, overlook the true variability of AIDS."

Dr. Maureen Goodenov remarks on this new finding: "Virologists are still underestimating the variability of these viruses. Every virus is unique, every viral genome is unique, and every group of viruses isolated from the body appears to be a mixture of viruses."

One of the great concerns that epidemiologists have about AIDS is the long incubation period in which patients can be entirely asymptomatic but be carrying the deadly infectious virus.

Perhaps the most shocking news that came out of the Stockholm meeting has received the least amount of press. Dr Alvaro Muñoz of Johns Hopkins University suggested that the median AIDS-free time *before seroconversion* may be 14 years. (Seroconversion means a positive blood test).

At this same meeting it was reported that some patients may go as long as four years from the time of infection until their blood seroconverts. This would indicate that it is possible for a patient to go as long as *18 years* before being diagnosed and showing symptoms of the AIDS disease.[7]

Researchers have discovered that the AIDS virus can prevent antibodies from attacking it by simply changing one amino acid on its surface. The scientist reporting this startling finding said, "This is one of the worst possible scenarios" for developing an AIDS vaccine.

The AIDS virus frequently mutates, and so a neutralizing antibody developed against one genetic strain of AIDS will not work against a second strain. It appears that each AIDS patient is harboring a slightly different virus, and therefore it will probably be necessary to *develop a different vaccine for each and every patient.* It has also been found that the AIDS strain in a particular patient gets more virulent with time. This was proven by making cultures periodically and, in most cases, the AIDS virus is more potent each time it is checked.

Adding to this depressing news, Dr. Michael G. Koch of Sweden confirmed that a long latency period between infection and evidence of the virus in the blood was not unusual. This means that a person can be harboring the AIDS virus and the blood test will not reveal it for long periods of time, thereby causing widespread dissemination of the disease by a person not knowing that he has AIDS.

Dr. José González reported in New Scientist magazine on the 14th of July, 1988 that the delay in the spread of AIDS will be 10 times the latency period. That is, if the period between infection and the blood test becoming positive is one year, then it would take ten years for the spread of the disease to be manifest. This means that tens

---

7 *Internal Medicine News,* August 1-14. 1988.

of millions of people could now be infected and not know it. It may be another 10, 20 or even 30 years before we'll know the true extent of the AIDS epidemic.

It is highly significant that the AIDS virus is very similar morphologically, biologically and molecularly to the sheep visna virus, the equine infectious anemia virus and the feline immuno-deficiency virus. It also has some characteristics of the bovine leukemia virus. The CD-4 molecule is the high affinity receptor for the HIV virus.[8] After the HIV virus connects with the CD-4 molecule, the virus is brought into the cell and loses its sugar coat.

Once brought into the cell the genomic RNA is transcribed by the use of the enzyme reverse transcriptase to DNA, and this new DNA form of the AIDS virus is integrated into the chromosomes of the receptor cell.

When the virus replicates itself within the T-cells the host T-cell is usually killed. However, this does not usually happen with the macrophages. The macrophage may simply harbor the virus in a quiescent state or it may produce a massive amount of virus which it holds for an indeterminate length of time without actually killing the macrophage. The T-8 cells, like the macrophage, seem to be free of any cytopathic effect from the HIV virus.

One of the mysteries of AIDS is the difficulty in explaining why the T-cells are so dramatically affected when such a small number of them are actually destroyed by the AIDS virus. Far less than one-tenth of one percent of the circulating T-cells are involved when the peripheral blood is tested. However, it is believed that many more may be involved, but are not expressing this through known testing methods.

It is also possible that T-4 precursor or stem cells are infected so fewer T-cells are produced, therefore decreasing the overall number of circulating T-4 cells.

---

8 Dalgleish, et. al., *Nature*: 312-763 (1984).

The reason the T-4 cells are so critical and a reduction in their overall number leads to disaster for the patient is because of the remarkable number of roles that the T-4 lymphocyte plays in the overall immunological defenses of the body. As the pituitary is a master gland, the T-4 certainly is a master lymphocyte.

The T-4s, either directly or indirectly, do all of the following:

1) Activate macrophages
2) Secrete growth factors for lymphoid cells
3) Secrete hematopoetic colony-stimulating factors
4) Secrete factors which induce non-lymphoid cell function
5) Induce B-cell function
6) Induce suppressor cell function
7) Induce N-K cell function
8) Induce cytotoxic T-cell function

Like oxygen, water and food, T-4 cells are essential to life.

Probably the main reason AIDS patients are so susceptible to pyogenic infections is because of the action of the T-cells on B-cells. The pathogenic B-cell leads to a deficiency in antibody response to antigens such as pyogenic bacteria. This sick B-cell condition also causes a high incidence of Epstein-Barr (EBV) and Cytomegalovirus (CMV) in these patients.

Also, paradoxically, although the number of circulating natural killer (NK) cells is not significantly diminished in the AIDS-infected individual, and these cells continue to bind normally to their target cells, they are not effective in their ability to kill.

Although the T-cell appears to be the central problem in lack of resistance to infection in AIDS, an even greater enemy turns out to be the "treason of the macrophage." They play a major role in the pathogenesis and propagation of AIDS infection because they engulf the virus, store them and reproduce them. One of the few cells to penetrate the blood/brain barrier is the macrophage, consequently the macrophage carries the HIV infection directly to the brain. Changes in mentation and severe psychiatric disturbances follow.

The macrophage also carries the AIDS virus into the bone where it can simply dock and remain quiescent for years. As the monocyte (macrophage) is refractory to the toxic effects of HIV, the virus can survive and replicate for an indefinite period of time. It is now believed that the main reason AIDS-infected patients check out negative on the AIDS test is because the virus is hiding in these macrophages which have been docked in the central nervous system and in the bone.

Another disturbing aspect of this "treason of the macrophage" is that these cells are found in every layer of the skin. The virus is right at the surface within these macrophages and so subject to spread from person to person through cuts on the skin. The virus is also readily available to blood sucking insects such as mosquitoes, bed bugs, ticks, fleas and others

There is a question as to how the macrophage can contain the virus and yet go months or even years without reproducing within its body. The most likely scenario is that two integrated copies of pro-virus are in each cell and are simply waiting to be called. It is believed that certain cytokines are responsible for this triggering of the growth of the virus within the macrophage. This induction may be caused by syphilis, herpes, Epstein-Barr virus or many other suspected co-factors.

It is significant that AIDS infection of macrophages does not cause a pathogenic reponse in this particular cell. This is analogous to infection with the other lente viruses such as the sheep visna virus, the equine infectious anemia virus and the caprine encephalitis-arthritis virus of goats. In these lente viruses,* as in HIV, there is an ineffective immune response and therefore it is often impossible to have an effective immune surveillance.

Dr. Peter Duesberg, famous for saying that the AIDS virus doesn't cause AIDS because it does not fill Koch's postulates, should note carefully that (1) Koch's postulates have been discredited and (2) even if you do believe that Koch's postulates must be fulfilled to prove an infecting agent, it may simply be that the virus is in hiding and therefore Koch's postulates cannot be fulfilled until the virus is good and ready. Dr. Duesberg has said that he is so certain that the AIDS virus does not cause AIDS that he would be willing to inject himself with AIDS virus. I doubt that he will do this.

In summary:
1. Susceptible monocytes/macrophages survive infection with the HIV virus and are either latently infected with the integrated pro-virus without virus expression or chronically infected with very, very low virus production within the cell.
2. It appears certain that activation signals are required for the establishment of HIV infection from these cells.
3. HIV infection can obviously live for prolonged periods of time latently or in chronic form in macrophages and monocytes. Activation signals or "co-factors" are necessary to convert a latent or chronic infection to an overt clinical AIDS infection

AIDS-Induced Brain Disease (AIBD)

It is now clear that AIDS causes a direct infection of the brain. Undoubtedly it is carried across the blood/brain barrier in the macrophage. After entering the brain these infected cells release enzymes that are toxic to neurons and hence cause a toxic reaction such as any toxin

---

*The lente viruses arc slow-acting retroviruses, like AIDS.

247

could cause in any other area of the body such as the plague bacillus toxin or the toxin of anthrax.

Recent research[9] indicates that the AIDS virus directly infects the neurons and glial cells just as it infects T-4 cells and monocytes. Also GP-120 protein of the AIDS virus envelope inhibits the growth of nerve cells.

RECOMMENDED READING:

Fauci, "The Human Immunodeficiency Virus: Infectivity and Mechanism of Pathogenesis," *Science*, 2/5/88.

"Viruses Work to Improve Their Image," *New Scientist*, 5/19/88.

Joklik, **Virology**, second edition.

Strecker, *The Strecker Memorandum*, available on the internet by searching for keywords: "Strecker Memorandum"

---

9   Wiley, et. al., *Proc. Nail. Acad. Sci*, 83,7089, (1986).

Chapter 13
What Can We Do?

The answer to a defense against AIDS is not antibiotics and it is not vaccines. Clearly vaccines have been proven to be of little effectiveness, even against "ordinary" germs. In the case of these new recombinant agents, they would be totally ineffective—the germs would be designed to be vaccine-proof.

The answer lies in photophoretic and electromagnetic medicine. The photophoretic method would be the simplest and therefore the most practical. We will need a virtual army of "photophoretic technicians" to protect troops and civilian populations alike (see next page).

The American military is finally awakening to the devastating and shocking threat of biological weapons. Plans are now afoot to protect the American military, but there are no plans to do anything to protect the civilian population of the United States. In other words, *you are on your own.*

So what can we do?

Every family is going to have to build its own medical moat. This medical moat will consist of certain key antibiotics, pharmaceuticals and an ultra-violet photophoresis instrument.

The antibiotics needed are chloromycetin (chloramphenocol) for intravenous administration; streptomycin, also for intravenous use; and some form of tetracycline for oral use. Penicillin should also be available. Penicillin will be only a secondary drug as a defense against biological warfare. Most of the agents likely to be used will not respond to penicillin—plague bacillus and anthrax, for examples.

The organo-phosphates maybe employed in a chemical attack, although I do not anticipate that they will be major weapons as they are "one time only" agents. They do not spread from person to person. However, a complete biochemical warfare kit should contain injectable atropine for protection against these chemical compounds.

By far the most important tool for biological defense is the photophoretic instrument mentioned above. Photo refers to light, and phoresis refers to drawing out of blood. A small amount of blood is withdrawn from a vein. This blood is put into a ultra-violet light machine of a set frequency for a measured period of time. This blood is then reinjected into the patient. An immediate and dramatic stimulation of the immune system occurs. Toxins such as cobra and spider venom, botulinum toxin and the toxin of plague are instantly neutralized. The treatment also destroys viruses, bacteria, protozoa and fungi very quickly. This machine, with our current available technology, is our best hope of surviving a bio attack.

Every household needs to have a designated biological defense person. This family member is trained to draw blood and to set up intravenous fluids as for the administration of antibiotics. He would also be in charge of the photophoretic equipment. You cannot depend on government agencies, including the military, to protect you against biological attack. You should prepare your family now while there is still time.

The *New York Times* (4/23/84) reports: "The worst fears of molecular biologists may soon be realized. A seven month investigation by the *Wall Street Journal* reveals that the Soviet Union is engaged in an intensive research program focused on using the revolutionary techniques of recombinant DNA to create a new generation of germ warfare agents."

The future is indeed grim, and only those who are prepared will survive.

Action needed now:

1. Immediately stop all illegal entry into the United States, especially that from Mexico, by using whatever means necessary. Not only AIDS, but illegal drugs are flooding this nation from across the Mexican border. We must clearly recognize this as war and an invasion with deadly weapons. Unfortunately, many innocent Mexicans will suffer from this interdiction. But we are talking national survival and we must, at least this once, place our interests above others.

2. Immediately close down all bath houses and pornography shops where people involved in various types of aberrant sex are prone to gather.

3. Severely punish children involved in sexual and drug activity in the schools.

4. Stop all school-sponsored sex education which is working against the best interests of our children. We have had a dramatic increase in venereal disease and pregnancy in our country during the 20 years of so-called "sex education."

5. We must immediately test all Americans for AIDS from birth onward. The AIDS-infected must understand that it will be a criminal offense to have sex or do anything else that tends to spread the AIDS epidemic, such as working in restaurants, hospitals and other places with a close association with

251

uninfected people.

6. We recommend, until the epidemic is brought under control, that you remove your children from school and teach them at home. If you do not feel comfortable with this, perhaps you can join with a few other families to spread the responsibility. The schools are rapidly becoming an important nidus of infection and the schools may have to be temporarily closed.

7. All AIDS-positive prostitutes, male and female, should be incarcerated for life or until an AIDS cure is discovered.

8. As narcotic drug abuse is an important avenue of transmission of the AIDS virus, we should impose the death penalty on all purveyors and, if that is not effective, on users of hard drugs.

9. You should avoid mosquitoes and insect-infested areas.

10. It is important that the home be kept immaculately clean and all family members physically clean. One of the greatest advances in public health has been the elimination of filth which is prone to spread all diseases. It is certainly possible that bed bugs, roaches, fleas, ticks, mosquitoes and other insects, both blood-sucking and non-blood-sucking, may now or in the future play a role in the spread of the AIDS virus. Cleanliness is of paramount importance (especially when living under crowded conditions).

11. Find a doctor who is not afraid to try innovative methods of treatment such as hydrogen peroxide, photophoresis, mega-vitamin therapy, chelation

and, once it is available, the Rife ray therapy.

12. Prisoners with AIDS who have any history of violence, whether related to their conviction or not, should remain in prison until a cure for AIDS is discovered.

13. We must investigate vigorously the Rife ray, the Tesla method, the Antoine Prioré method, and the electromagnetic device of Professor Wollin. *All these various electro-magnetic and photoelectric therapies have been proven to cure cancer* and will, if not cure AIDS, at least give us methods to bring it under control until a cure can be found.

14. We must lobby vigorously, on both state and federal levels, if any definitive remedy is to be found. Congress must put the Soviet Union and the narcotic-producing countries on notice that biological and drug sabotage will no longer be tolerated. In a free nation the political process works to our advantage. It is truly a gift of God that we must take advantage of. Our representatives act only if we demand it. This strong political action to bring an implementation of all the above recommendations must be accomplished soon or the game is indeed lost.

***

We may have to return to a very rigid standard of conduct backed by law and penalties for misconduct. We need to study carefully the great plagues and the social upheaval they caused because the situation today is parallel. As plagues are spread more rapidly through close association of people, licentiousness and general debauchery tend to spread the disease. This was quite evident during the plague years. It contributed to an already serious situation.

If this were to happen today, and all caution were

thrown to the winds due to the attitude that the situation is hopeless and "I might as well get what I can," it would only compound an already deadly trend.

This is illustrated very clearly from reports of the plague years:

"Men resolved to get out of life the pleasures which could be had speedily and would satisfy their lusts, regarding their bodies and their wealth alike as transitory . . . no fear of gods or law of men restrained them; for, on the one hand, seeing that all men were perishing alike, they judged that piety or impiety came to the same thing, and, on the other hand, no one expected that he would live to be called to account and pay the penalty for his misdeeds. On the contrary, they believed that the penalty already decreed against them and now hanging over their heads was a far heavier one, and that before it fell it was only reasonable to get some enjoyment out of life."[1]

A similar reaction occurred 1700 years later proving that human nature indeed does not change. People in England gave themselves up to carousing and drinking during the plagues of the Middle Ages.

Theologian John Wycliffe wrote in the 14th century with dismay of the lawlessness and depravity of the time. Chroniclers reported there was "drinking, roaring and surfeiting... in one house you might hear them roaring under the pangs of death, and in the next tippling, roaring and belching out blasphemies against God."

With these historical precedents, it appears that regulation of social behavior, as much as we hate it in an egalitarian society such as ours, may be necessary for the survival of our civilization. Most are not going to like it, especially those who are involved in casual sex, recreational use of drugs and the other by-products of our open society.

---

1   Thucidides, **Plague** of Athens, 430 B.C

About Doctor William Campbell Douglass II

Dr. Douglass reveals medical truths, and deceptions, often at risk of being labeled heretical. He is consumed by a passion for living a long healthy life, and wants his readers to share that passion. Their health and well-being comes first. He is anti-dogmatic, and unwavering in his dedication to improve the quality of life of his readers. He has been called "the conscience of modern medicine," a "medical maverick," and has been voted "Doctor of the Year" by the National Health Federation. His medical experiences are far reaching-from battling malaria in Central America - to fighting deadly epidemics at his own health clinic in Africa - to flying with U.S. Navy crews as a flight surgeon - to working for 10 years in emergency medicine here in the States. These learning experiences, not to mention his keen storytelling ability and wit, make Dr. Douglass' newsletters (Daily Dose and Real Health) and books uniquely interesting and fun to read. He shares his no-frills, no-bull approach to health care, often amazing his readers by telling them to ignore many widely-hyped good-health practices (like staying away from red meat, avoiding coffee, and eating like a bird), and start living again by eating REAL food, taking some inexpensive supplements, and doing the pleasurable things that make life livable. Readers get all this, plus they learn how to burn fat, prevent cancer, boost libido, and so much more. And, Dr. Douglass is not afraid to challenge the latest studies that come out, and share the real story with his readers. Dr. William C. Douglass has led a colorful, rebellious, and crusading life. Not many physicians would dare put their professional reputations on the line as many times as this courageous healer has. A vocal opponent of "business-as-usual" medicine, Dr. Douglass has championed patients' rights and physician commitment to wellness throughout his career. This dedicated physician has repeatedly gone far beyond the call of duty in his work to spread the truth about alternative therapies. For a full year, he endured economic and physical hardship to work with physicians at the Pasteur Institute in St. Petersburg, Russia, where advanced research on photoluminescence was being conducted. Dr. Douglass comes from a distinguished family of physicians. He is the fourth generation Douglass to practice medicine, and his son is also a physician. Dr. Douglass graduated from the University of Rochester, the Miami School of Medicine, and the Naval School of Aviation and Space Medicine.

You want to protect those you love from the health dangers the authorities aren't telling you about, and learn the incredible cures that they've scorned and ignored?

Subscribe to the free Daily Dose updates "...the straight scoop about health, medicine, and politics." by sending an e-mail to real_sub@agoramail.net with the word "subscribe" in the subject line.

Dr. William Campbell Douglass'
Real Health:

Had Enough?

Enough turkey burgers and sprouts?

Enough forcing gallons of water down your throat?

Enough exercising until you can barely breathe?

Before you give up everything just because "everyone" says it's healthy...

Learn the facts from Dr. William Campbell Douglass, medicine's most acclaimed myth-buster. In every issue of Dr. Douglass' Real Health newsletter, you'll learn shocking truths about "junk medicine" and how to stay healthy while eating eggs, meat and other foods you love.

With the tips you'll receive from Real Health, you'll see your doctor less, spend a lot less money and be happier and healthier while you're at it. The road to Real Health is actually easier, cheaper and more pleasant than you dared to dream.

*Subscribe to Real Health today by calling 1-800-981-7162 or visit the Real Health web site at www.realhealthnews.com.
Use promotional code : DRHBDZZZ*

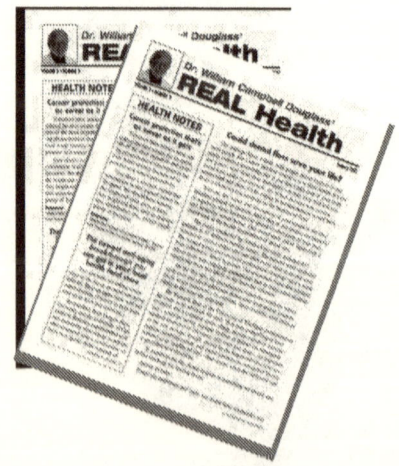

If you knew of a procedure that could save thousands, maybe millions, of people dying from AIDS, cancer, and other dreaded killers....

Would you cover it up?

It's unthinkable that what could be the best solution ever to stopping the world's killer diseases is being ignored, scorned, and rejected. But that is exactly what's happening right now.

The procedure is called "photoluminescence". It's a thoroughly tested, proven therapy that uses the healing power of the light to perform almost miraculous cures.

This remarkable treatment works its incredible cures by stimulating the body's own immune responses. That's why it cures so many ailments--and why it's been especially effective against AIDS! Yet, 50 years ago, it virtually disappeared from the halls of medicine.

Why has this incredible cure been ignored by the medical authorities of this country? You'll find the shocking answer here in the pages of this new edition of Into the Light. Now available with the blood irradiation Instrument Diagram and a complete set of instructions for building your own "Treatment Device". Also includes details on how to use this unique medical instrument.

Into the Light

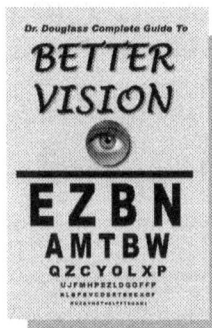

Dr. Douglass' Complete Guide to Better Vision

A report about eyesight and what can be done to improve it naturally. But I've also included information about how the eye works, brief descriptions of various common eye conditions, traditional remedies to eye problems, and a few simple suggestions that may help you maintain your eyesight for years to come.
-William Campbell Douglass II, MD

The Hypertension Report.
Say Good Bye to High Blood Pressure.

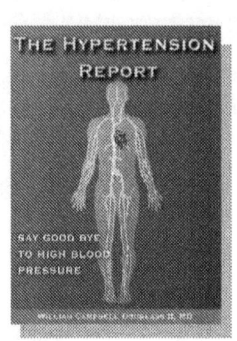

An estimated 50 million Americans have high blood pressure. Often called the "silent killer" because it may not cause symptoms until the patient has suffered serious damage to the arterial system. Diet, exercise, potassium supplements chelation therapy and practically anything but drugs is the way to go and alternatives are discussed in this report.

Grandma Bell's A To Z Guide To Healing With Herbs.

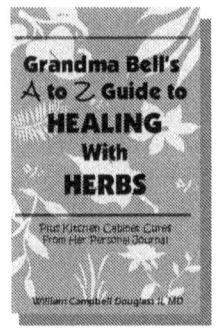

This book is all about - coming home. What I once believed to be old wives' tales - stories long destroyed by the new world of science - actually proved to be the best treatment for many of the common ailments you and I suffer through. So I put a few of them together in this book with the sincere hope that Grandma Bell's wisdom will help you recover your common sense, and take responsibility for your own health. -William Campbell Douglass II, MD

Prostate Problems:
Safe, Simple, Effective Relief for Men over 50.

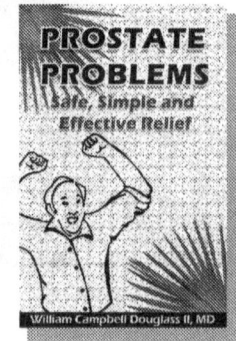

Don't be frightened into surgery or drugs you may not need. First, get the facts about prostate problems... know all your options, so you can make the best decisions. This fully documented report explains the dangers of conventional treatments, and gives you alternatives that could save you more than just money!

Color me Healthy
The Healing Powers of Colors

"He's crazy!"
"He's got to be a quack!"
"Who gave this guy his medical license?"
"He's a nut case!"

In case you're wondering, those are the reactions you'll probably get if you show your doctor this report. I know the idea of healing many common ailments simply by exposing them to colored light sounds far-fetched, but when you see the evidence, you'll agree that color is truly an amazing medical breakthrough.

When I first heard the stories, I reacted much the same way. But the evidence so convinced me, that I had to try color therapy in my practice. My results were truly amazing.

-William Campbell Douglass II, MD

Order your complete set of Roscolene filters (choice of 3 sizes) to be used with the "Color Me Healthy" therapy. The eleven Roscolene filters are # 809, 810, 818, 826, 828, 832, 859, 861, 866, 871, and 877. The filters come with protective separator sheets between each filter. The color names and the Roscolene filter(s) used to produce that particular color, are printed on a card included with the filters and a set of instructions on how to fit them to a lamp.

What Is Going on Here?

Peroxides are supposed to be bad for you. Free radicals and all that. But now we hear that hydrogen peroxide is good for us. Hydrogen peroxide will put extra oxygen in your blood. There's no doubt about that. Hydrogen peroxide costs pennies. So if you can get oxygen into the blood cheaply and safely, maybe cancer (which doesn't like oxygen), emphysema, AIDS, and many other terrible diseases can be treated effectively. Intravenous hydrogen peroxide rapidly relieves allergic reactions, influenza symptoms, and acute viral infections.

No one expects to live forever. But we would all like to have a George Burns finish. The prospect of finishing life in a nursing home after abandoning your tricycle in the mobile home park is not appealing. Then comes the loss of control of vital functions the ultimate humiliation. Is life supposed to be from tricycle to tricycle and diaper to diaper? You come into this world crying, but do you have to leave crying? I don't believe you do. And you won't either after you see the evidence. Sounds too good to be true, doesn't it? Read on and decide for yourself.

-William Campbell Douglass II, MD

Rhino Publishing S.A.
www.rhinopublish.com

HYDROGEN PEROXIDE

Medical Miracle

H_2O

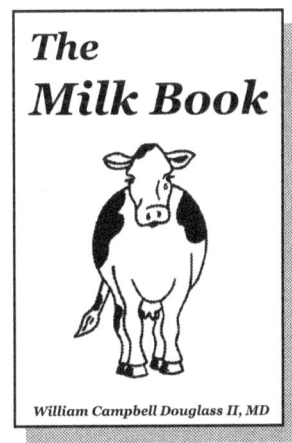

Eat Your Cholesterol!
Eat Meat, Drink Milk, Spread The Butter- And Live Longer!
How to Live off the Fat of the Land and Feel Great.

Americans are being saturated with anti-cholesterol propaganda. If you watch very much television, you're probably one of the millions of Americans who now has a terminal case of cholesterol phobia. The propaganda is relentless and is often designed to produce fear and loathing of this worst of all food contaminants. You never hear the food propagandists bragging about their product being fluoride-free or aluminum-free, two of our truly serious food-additive problems. But cholesterol, an essential nutrient, not proven to be harmful in any quantity, is constantly pilloried as a menace to your health. If you don't use corn oil, Fleischmann's margarine, and Egg Beaters, you're going straight to atherosclerosis hell with stroke, heart attack, and premature aging -- and so are your kids. Never feel guilty about what you eat again! Dr. Douglass shows you why red meat, eggs, and dairy products aren't the dietary demons we're told they are. But beware: This scientifically sound report goes against all the "common wisdom" about the foods you should eat. Read with an open mind.

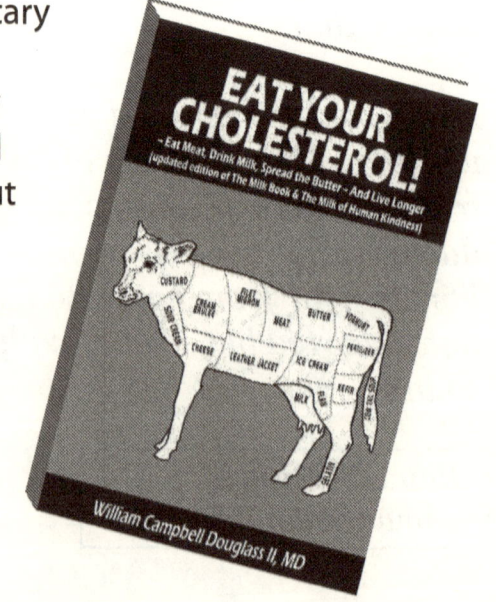

Rhino Publishing, S.A.
www.rhinopublish.com

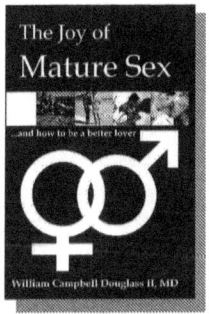

The Joy of Mature Sex and How to Be a Better Lover

Humans are very confused about what makes good sex. But I believe humans have more to offer each other than this total licentiousness common among animals. We're talking about mature sex. The kind of sex that made this country great.

Stop Aging or Slow the Process How Exercise With Oxygen Therapy (EWOT) Can Help

EWOT (pronounced ee-watt) stands for Exercise With Oxygen Therapy. This method of prolonging your life is so simple and you can do it at home at a minimal cost. When your cells don't get enough oxygen, they degenerate and die and so you degenerate and die. It's as simple as that.

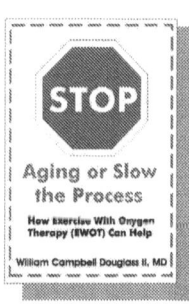

Hormone Replacement Therapies: Astonishing Results For Men And Women

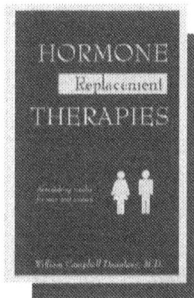

It is accurate to say that when the endocrine glands start to fail, you start to die. We are facing a sea change in longevity and health in the elderly. Now, with the proper supplemental hormones, we can slow the aging process and, in many cases, reverse some of the signs and symptoms of aging.

Add 10 Years to Your Life With some "best of" Dr. Douglass' writings.

To add ten years to your life, you need to have the right attitude about health and an understanding of the health industry and what it's feeding you. Following the established line on many health issues could make you very sick or worse! Achieve dynamic health with this collection of some of the "best of" Dr. Douglass' newsletters.

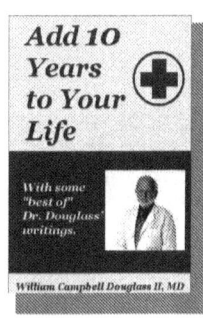

PAINFUL DILEMMA

Are we fighting the wrong war?

We are spending millions on the war against drugs while we
should be fighting the war against pain with those drugs!

As you will read in this book, the war on drugs was lost a long time ago and,
when it comes to the war against pain, pain is winning! An article in USA Today
(11/20/02) reveals that dying patients are not getting relief from pain. It seems
the doctors are torn between fear of the government, certainly justified, and a
clinging to old and out dated ideas about pain, which is NOT justified.

A group called Last Acts, a coalition of health-care groups, has released a very
discouraging study of all 50 states that nearly half of the 1.6 million Americans
living in nursing homes suffer from untreated pain. They said that life was being
extended but it amounted to little more than "extended pain and suffering."

This book offers insight into the history of pain treatment and the current failed
philosophies of contemporary medicine. Plus it describes some of today's most
advanced treatments for alleviating certain kinds of pain. This book is not another
"self-help" book touting home remedies; rather, Painful Dilemma: Patients in
Pain -- People in Prison, takes a hard look at where we've gone wrong and what
we (you) can do to help a loved one who is living with chronic pain.

The second half of this book is a must read if you value your freedom. We now
have the ridiculous and tragic situation of people
in pain living in a government-created hell by
restriction of narcotics and people in prison for
trying to bring pain relief by the selling of
narcotics to the suffering. The end result of the
"war on drugs" has been to create the greatest
and most destructive cartel in history, so great,
in fact, that the drug Mafia now controls most
of the world economy.

Rhino Publishing S.A.
www.rhinopublish.com

Live the Adventure!

Why would anyone in their right mind put everything they own in storage and move to Russia, of all places?! But when maverick physician Bill Douglass left a profitable medical practice in a peaceful mountaintop town to pursue "pure medical truth".... none of us who know him well was really surprised.

After All, anyone who's braved the outermost reaches of darkest Africa, the mean streets of Johannesburg and New York, and even a trip to Washington to testify before the Senate, wouldn't bat and eye at ducking behind the Iron Curtain for a little medical reconnaissance!

Enjoy this imaginative, funny, dedicated man's tales of wonder and woe as he treks through a year in St. Petersburg, working on a cure for the world's killer diseases. We promise --

YOU WON'T BE BORED!

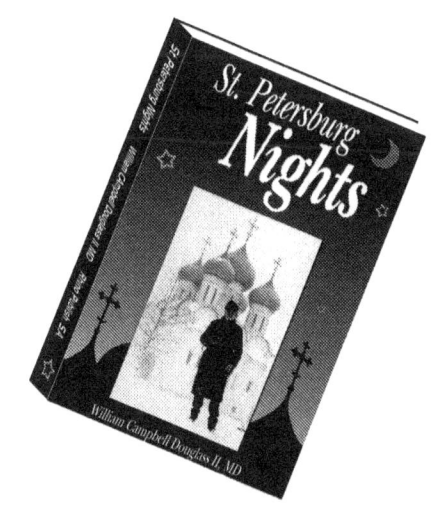

Rhino Publishing S.A.
www.rhinopublish.com

THE SMOKER'S PARADOX
THE HEALTH BENEFITS OF TOBACCO!

The benefits of smoking tobacco have been common knowledge for centuries. From sharpening mental acuity to maintaining optimal weight, the relatively small risks of smoking have always been outweighed by the substantial improvement to mental and physical health. Hysterical attacks on tobacco notwithstanding, smokers always weigh the good against the bad and puff away or quit according to their personal preferences. Now the same anti-tobacco enterprise that has spent billions demonizing the pleasure of smoking is providing additional reasons to smoke. Alzheimer's, Parkinson's, Tourette's Syndrome, even schizophrenia and cocaine addiction are disorders that are alleviated by tobacco. Add in the still inconclusive indication that tobacco helps to prevent colon and prostate cancer and the endorsement for smoking tobacco by the medical establishment is good news for smokers and non-smokers alike. Of course the revelation that tobacco is good for you is ruined by the pharmaceutical industry's plan to substitute the natural and relatively inexpensive tobacco plant with their overpriced and ineffective nicotine substitutions. Still, when all is said and done, the positive revelations regarding tobacco are very good reasons indeed to keep lighting those cigars - but only 4 a day!

Rhino Publishing, S.A
www.rhinopublish.com

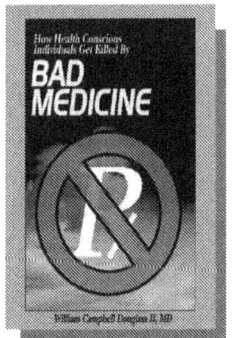

Bad Medicine
How Individuals Get Killed By Bad Medicine.

Do you really need that new prescription or that overnight stay in the hospital? In this report, Dr. Douglass reveals the common medical practices and misconceptions endangering your health. Best of all, he tells you the pointed (but very revealing!) questions your doctor prays you never ask. Interesting medical facts about popular remedies are revealed.

Dangerous Legal Drugs
The Poisons in Your Medicine Chest.

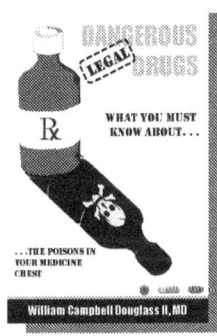

If you knew what we know about the most popular prescription and over-the-counter drugs, you'd be sick. That's why Dr. Douglass wrote this shocking report about the poisons in your medicine chest. He gives you the low-down on different categories of drugs. Everything from painkillers and cold remedies to tranquilizers and powerful cancer drugs.

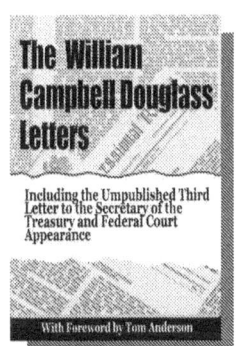

The William Campbell Douglass Letters.
Expose of Government Machinations
(Vietnam War).

THE WILLIAM CAMPBELL DOUGLASS LETTERS. Dr. Douglass' Defense in 1968 Tax Case and Expose of Government Machinations during the Vietnam War.

The Eagle's Feather. A Novel of
International Political Intrigue.

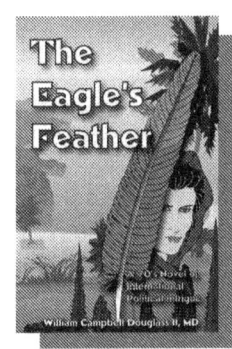

Although The Eagle's Feather is a work of fiction set in the 1970's, it is built, as with most fiction, on a framework of plausibility and background information. This is a fiction book that could not have been written were it not for various ominous aspects, which pose a clear and present danger to the security of the United States.

Rhino
Publishing

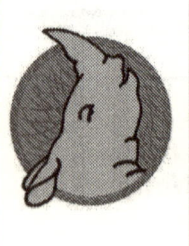

ORDER
FORM

PURCHASER INFORMATION

Purchaser's Name (Please Print): _____

Shipping Address (Do not use a P.O. Box): _____

City: _____ State/Prov.: _____ Country: _____

Zip/Postal Code: _____ Telephone No.: _____ Fax No.: _____

E-Mail Address (if interested in receiving free e-Books when available): _____

CREDIT CARD INFO (CIRCLE ONE):

MASTERCARD, VISA, AMERICAN EXPRESS, DISCOVER, JCB, DINER'S CLUB, CARTE BLANCHE.

Charge my Card -> Number #: _____ Exp.: _____

*Security Code: _____ * Required for all MasterCard, Visa and American Express purchases. For your security, we require that you enter your card's verification number. The verification number is also called a CCV number. This code is the 3 digits farthest right in the signature field on the back of your VISA/MC, or the 4 digits to the right on the front of your American Express card. Your credit card statement will show **a different name than Rhino Publishing** as the vendor.

WE DO NOT share your private information, we use 3rd party credit card processing service to process your order only.

ADDITIONAL INFORMATION

If your shipping address is not the same as your credit card billing address, please indicate your card billing address here.

Name on the card _____ Type of card: _____

Billing Address: _____

City: _____ State/Prov.: _____ Zip/Postal Code: _____

Fax a copy of this order to:
RHINO PUBLISHING, S.A.
1-888-317-6767 or International #: + 416-352-5126

To order by mail, send your payment by first class mail only to the following address. Please include a copy of this order form. Make your check or bank drafts (NO postal money order) payable to RHINO PUBLISHING, S.A. and mail to:

Rhino Publishing, S.A.
Attention: PTY 5048
P.O. Box 025724
Miami, FL.
USA 33102

Digital E-books also available online: www.rhinopublish.com

Rhino Publishing

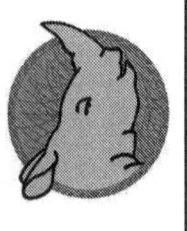

ORDER FORM

Purchaser's Name (Please Print): _____

I would like to order the following paperback book of Dr. Douglass (Alternative Medicine Books):

___ X ___	9962-636-04-3	Add 10 Years to Your Life. With some "best of" Dr. Douglass writings.	$13.99 $____
___ X ___	9962-636-07-8	AIDS and Biological Warfare. What They Are Not Telling You!	$17.99 $____
___ X ___	9962-636-09-4	Bad Medicine. How Individuals Get Killed By Bad Medicine.	$11.99 $____
___ X ___	9962-636-10-8	Color Me Healthy. The Healing Power of Colors.	$11.99 $____
___ X ___	9962-636 -XX-X	Color Filters for Color Me Healthy. 11 Basic Roscolene Filters for Lamps.	$21.89 $____
___ X ___	9962-636-15-9	Dangerous Legal Drugs. The Poisons in Your Medicine Chest.	$13.99 $____
___ X ___	9962-636-18-3	Dr. Douglass' Complete Guide to Better Vision. Improve eyesight naturally.	$11.99 $____
___ X ___	9962-636-19-1	Eat Your Cholesterol! How to Live off the Fat of the Land and Feel Great.	$11.99 $____
___ X ___	9962-636-12-4	Grandma Bell's A To Z Guide To Healing. Her Kitchen Cabinet Cures.	$14.99 $____
___ X ___	9962-636-22-1	Hormone Replacement Therapies. Astonishing Results For Men & Women	$11.99 $____
___ X ___	9962-636-25-6	Hydrogen Peroxide: One of the Most Underused Medical Miracle.	$15.99 $____
___ X ___	9962-636-27-2	Into the Light. New Edition with Blood Irradiation Instrument Instructions.	$19.99 $____
___ X ___	9962-636-54-X	Milk Book. The Classic on the Nutrition of Milk and How to Benefit from it.	$17.99 $____

__ X	9962-636-00-0	Painful Dilemma - Patients in Pain - People in Prison.	$17.99 $ ___
__ X	9962-636-32-9	Prostate Problems. Safe, Simple, Effective Relief for Men over 50.	$11.99 $ ___
__ X	9962-636-34-5	St. Petersburg Nights. Enlightening Story of Life and Science in Russia.	$17.99 $ ___
__ X	9962-636-37-X	Stop Aging or Slow the Process. Exercise With Oxygen Therapy Can Help.	$11.99 $ ___
__ X	9962-636-60-4	The Hypertension Report. Say Good Bye to High Blood Pressure.	$11.99 $ ___
__ X	9962-636-48-5	The Joy of Mature Sex and How to Be a Better Lover...	$13.99 $ ___
__ X	9962-636-43-4	The Smoker's Paradox: Health Benefits of Tobacco.	$14.99 $ ___

Political Books:

__ X	9962-636-40-X	The Eagle's Feather. A 70's Novel of International Political Intrigue.	$15.99 $ ___
__ X	9962-636-46-9	The W. C. D. Letters. Expose of Government Machinations (Vietnam War).	$11.99 $ ___

SUB-TOTAL: $ ___

ADD $5.00 HANDLING FOR YOUR ORDER: $ 5.00 $ 5.00

__ X ADD $2.50 SHIPPING FOR EACH ITEM ON ORDER: $ 2.50 $ ___

NOTE THAT THE MINIMUM SHIPPING AND HANDLING IS $7.50 FOR 1 BOOK ($5.00 + $2.50)
For order shipped outside the US, add $5.00 per item

__ X ADD $5.00 S. & H. OR EACH ITEM ON ORDER (INTERNATIONAL ORDERS ONLY) $ 5.00 $ ___
Allow up to 21 days for delivery (we will call you about back orders if any)

TOTAL: $ ___

Fax a copy of this order to: 1-888-317-6767 or Int'l + 416-352-5126
or mail to: Rhino Publishing, S.A. Attention: PTY 5048 P.O. Box 025724, Miami, FL., 33102 USA
Digital E-books also available online: www.rhinopublish.com

www.ingramcontent.com/pod-product-compliance
Lightning Source LLC
Chambersburg PA
CBHW020439130626
46549CB00001B/210